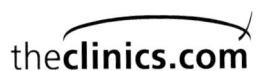

A. Simon Turner, BVSc, MS
CONSULTING EDITOR

VETERINARY CLINICS
OF NORTH AMERICA

Equine Practice

Urinary Tract Disorders

GUEST EDITOR
Harold C. Schott II, DVM, PhD

December 2007 • Volume 23 • Number 3

SAUNDERS

An Imprint of Elsevier, Inc.
PHILADELPHIA   LONDON   TORONTO   MONTREAL   SYDNEY   TOKYO

W.B. SAUNDERS COMPANY
A Division of Elsevier Inc.

Elsevier, Inc., 1600 John F. Kennedy Blvd., Suite 1800, Philadelphia, PA 19103-2899

http://www.vetequine.theclinics.com

VETERINARY CLINICS OF NORTH AMERICA:	**Volume 23, Number 3**
EQUINE PRACTICE	**ISSN 0749-0739**
December 2007	**ISBN-13: 978-1-4160-5134-3**
Editor: John Vassallo; j.vassallo@elsevier.com	**ISBN-10: 1-4160-5134-1**

The ideas and opinions expressed in *Veterinary Clinics of North America: Equine Practice* do not necessarily reflect those of the Publisher. The Publisher does not assume any responsibility for any injury and/or damage to persons or property arising out of or related to any use of the material contained in this periodical. The reader is advised to check the appropriate medical literature and the product information currently provided by the manufacturer of each drug to be administered to verify the dosage, the method and duration of administration, or contraindications. It is the responsibility of the treating physician or other health care professional, relying on independent experience and knowledge of the patient, to determine drug dosages and the best treatment for the patient. Mention of any product in this issue should not be construed as endorsement by the contributors, editors, or the Publisher of the product or manufacturers' claims.

Veterinary Clinics of North America: Equine Practice (ISSN 0749-0739) is published in April, August, and December by Elsevier Inc., 360 Park Avenue South, New York, NY 10010-1710. Business and Editorial Offices: 1600 John F. Kennedy Blvd., Suite 1800, Philadelphia, PA 19103-2899. Customer Service office: 6277 Sea Harbor Drive, Orlando, FL 32887-4800. Subscription prices are $182.00 per year for US individuals, $302.00 per year for US institutions, $91.00 per year for US students and residents, $212.00 per year for Canadian individuals, $369.00 per year for Canadian institutions, $230.00 per year for international individuals, $369.00 per year for international institutions and $116.00 per year for Canadian and foreign students/residents. To receive student/resident rate, orders must be accompanied by name of affiliated institution, date of term, and the *signature* of program/residency coordinator on institution letterhead. Orders will be billed at individual rate until proof of status is received. Foreign air speed delivery is included in all *Clinics* subscription prices. All prices are subject to change without notice. **POSTMASTER:** Send address changes to *Veterinary Clinics of North America: Equine Practice*, Elsevier Periodicals Customer Service, 6277 Sea Harbor Drive, Orlando, FL 32887-4800, USA; phone: 1-800-654-2452 [toll free number for US customers], or 1-407-345-4000 [customers outside US]; fax: 1-407-363-1354; e-mail: usjcs@elsevier.com.

Reprints. For copies of 100 or more, of articles in this publication, please contact the Commercial Reprints Department, Elsevier Inc., 360 Park Avenue South, New York, New York 10010-1710. Tel. (212) 633-3813, Fax: (212) 462-1935 e-mail: reprints@elsevier.com.

Veterinary Clinics of North America: Equine Practice is covered in *Index Medicus, Excerpta Medica, Current Contents/Agriculture, Biology and Environmental Sciences, and ISI.*

Printed in the United States of America.

CONSULTING EDITOR

A. SIMON TURNER, BVSc, MS, Diplomate, American College of Veterinary Surgeons; Professor, Department of Clinical Sciences, College of Veterinary Medicine and Biomedical Sciences, Colorado State University, Fort Collins, Colorado

GUEST EDITOR

HAROLD C. SCHOTT II, DVM, PhD, Diplomate, American College of Veterinary Internal Medicine; Professor of Equine Medicine, Department of Large Animal Clinical Sciences, College of Veterinary Medicine, Michigan State University, East Lansing, Michigan

CONTRIBUTORS

LUIS G. ARROYO, DVM, DVSc, Department of Pathobiology, Ontario Veterinary College, University of Guelph, Guelph, Ontario, Canada

KRISTIN P. CHANEY, DVM, Clinical Instructor, Department of Large Animal Clinical Sciences, College of Veterinary Medicine, Michigan State University, East Lansing, Michigan

KATJA F. DUESTERDIECK-ZELLMER, DrMedVet, MS, PhD, Diplomate, American College of Veterinary Surgeons; Assistant Professor of Large Animal Surgery, Department of Clinical Sciences, College of Veterinary Medicine, Oregon State University, Corvallis, Oregon

RAYMOND J. GEOR, BVSc, MVSc, PhD, Diplomate, American College of Veterinary Internal Medicine; Paul Mellon Distinguished Chair; and Director of Research, Middleburg Agricultural Research and Extension (MARE) Center, College of Agriculture and Life Sciences, Virginia Tech, Middleburg; Professor, Large Animal Clinical Sciences, Virginia-Maryland Regional College of Veterinary Medicine, Virginia Polytechnic Institute and State University, Blacksburg, Virginia

ERICA C. McKENZIE, BSc, BVMS, PhD, Assistant Professor of Large Animal Medicine, Clinical Sciences Department, College of Veterinary Medicine, Oregon State University, Corvallis, Oregon

DAVID G. SCHMITZ, DVM, MS, Diplomate, American College of Veterinary Internal Medicine; Associate Professor of Medicine, Department of Veterinary Large Animal Clinical Sciences, College of Veterinary Medicine, Texas A&M University, College Station, Texas

HAROLD C. SCHOTT II, DVM, PhD, Diplomate, American College of Veterinary Internal Medicine; Professor of Equine Medicine, Department of Large Animal Clinical Sciences, College of Veterinary Medicine, Michigan State University, East Lansing, Michigan

JOHN SCHUMACHER, DVM, MS, Department of Clinical Sciences, College of Veterinary Medicine, Auburn University, Alabama

HENRY R. STÄMPFLI, DVM, DrMedVet, Diplomate, American College of Veterinary Internal Medicine; Department of Clinical Studies, Ontario Veterinary College, University of Guelph, Guelph, Ontario, Canada

RAMIRO E. TORIBIO, DVM, MS, PhD, Diplomate, American College of Veterinary Internal Medicine; Assistant Professor, College of Veterinary Medicine, The Ohio State University, Columbus, Ohio

M. EILIDH WILSON, BVMS, Equine Internal Medicine Resident, Department of Large Animal Clinical Sciences, Veterinary Medical Center, Michigan State University, East Lansing, Michigan

CONTENTS

largely supportive, including correction of fluid deficits and electrolyte and acid–base disturbances and treatment and reversal of the underlying cause. Use of dopamine and mannitol to promote renal blood flow and urine output is no longer recommended.

Chronic renal failure is a syndrome of progressive loss of renal function that results in loss of urinary concentrating ability, retention of nitrogenous and other metabolic end products, alterations in electrolyte and acid-base status, and dysfunction of several hormone systems. This article describes the prevalence, causes, clinical signs, diagnostic evaluation, and management of horses afflicted with chronic renal failure. It is hoped that this article illustrates that chronic renal failure, when detected in the earlier stages of disease, can be managed successfully in the short-term allowing owners to enjoy a period of time of ongoing productivity, performance, or companionship until loss of condition reaches the point that euthanasia becomes warranted.

The prevalence of equine urolithiasis has been estimated to be low. In horses with clinical signs of urolithiasis, uroliths are most commonly encountered in the urinary bladder, but it is not uncommon to detect uroliths in more than one location. The most common clinical signs for cystic calculi are urine scalding of the hind limbs, hematuria, tenesmus and dysuria. Numerous surgical techniques and approaches have been described for the treatment of urolithiasis in horses; however, independent of which approach is chosen, the goal should be to remove all calculi completely from the urinary tract, thus decreasing the chance of recurrence of urolithiasis. Laser lithotripsy and shock wave lithotripsy represent means to fragment uroliths with little morbidity, but limited availability of and costs associated with the equipment have precluded these technologies from being used more commonly in horses.

Renal tubular disorders have been sporadically reported in horses. Only three types of tubular defects have been recognized: (1) nephrogenic diabetes insipidus, attributable to unresponsiveness of the renal tubules to antidiuretic hormone; (2) distal renal tubular acidosis (RTA; type I); and (3) proximal RTA (type II). The following review focuses on RTA and nephrogenic diabetes insipidus.

FORTHCOMING ISSUES

RECENT ISSUES

The Clinics are now available online!

Access your subscription at:
www.theclinics.com

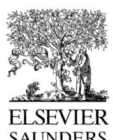

VETERINARY
CLINICS
Equine Practice

Vet Clin Equine 23 (2007) ix–x

Preface

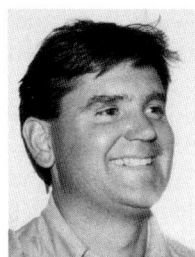

Harold C. Schott II, DVM, PhD
Guest Editor

The direction of many veterinarians' professional lives is strongly impacted by their early career experiences. This statement certainly holds true for my interest in urinary tract disorders in horses. During my first month in practice (more than 23 years ago), my early mentor (Richard Mansmann, VMD, PhD) and I were presented with a Saddlebred gelding at the National Horse and Flower Show in Santa Barbara, California, for evaluation of mild lethargy, a decreased appetite, and mild weight loss. Over the course of the next week we realized that the gelding was in end-stage chronic renal failure caused by glomerulonephritis. Another early case that further spurred my interest was an Arabian gelding that had three bouts of obstructive urethrolithiasis over several years; we ultimately determined this was a consequence of unilateral pyelonephritis. Renal ultrasonography and endoscopic examination of the urinary tract, with bilateral ureteral catheterization, were instrumental in finally establishing this diagnosis. After 3 years in private equine practice with Dr. Mansmann in Santa Barbara, I moved to academic practice (8 years at Washington State University and 12 years at Michigan State University) and have continued to maintain a strong interest in all things urinary.

Although generally considered uncommon, a wide range of equine urinary tract disorders can be presented to equine veterinarians. Many of these disorders are challenging to diagnose and manage, especially without use of high quality imaging devices (ultrasonography and endoscopy, in particular). In addition to just looking harder for problems of the urinary tract,

doi:10.1016/j.cveq.2007.11.001

I have gained clinical experience through long-term management of a number of patients with various problems over the years. In addition, I owe a debt of gratitude to the many practitioners with whom I have consulted over the past 20 years about urinary cases, and their willingness to provide me with follow-up information, as well as samples collected from their patients.

In this issue of *Veterinary Clinics of North America: Equine Practice*, I have been fortunate to gather a number of excellent equine clinicians to share their collective experience in the spectrum of urinary tract disorders. Some have presented their articles in the format of problems (eg, Polyuria and Polydipsia by McKenzie and Pigmenturia by Schumacher), while others have detailed disease syndromes (eg, Acute Renal Failure by Geor). To all authors, I extend my gratitude for your efforts in preparing up-to-date and practical information in your articles. It is the hope of all of the authors that this issue of *Clinics* will enable practitioners and students alike to approach horses with urinary tract disease in a more confident and focused direction and to provide an improved level of care to their patients.

Harold C. Schott II, DVM, PhD
Department of Large Animal Clinical Sciences
D-202 Veterinary Medical Center
Michigan State University
East Lansing, MI 48824-131, USA

E-mail address: schott@cvm.msu.edu

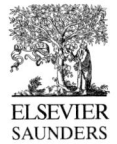

VETERINARY
CLINICS
Equine Practice

Vet Clin Equine 23 (2007) 533–561

Essentials of Equine Renal and Urinary Tract Physiology

Ramiro E. Toribio, DVM, MS, PhD

College of Veterinary Medicine, The Ohio State University,
601 Vernon Tharp Street, Columbus, OH 43210, USA

Understanding the basic aspects of urinary tract physiology is central to the clinical and therapeutic approach of various equine diseases. Knowledge of urinary tract anatomy and the numerous functions of the kidney in regulating fluids, electrolytes, acid-base balance, and waste products improves the ability of the clinician to diagnose, treat, and make appropriate recommendations for the management of the horse with renal disease. Several conditions can directly or indirectly affect renal function on a temporary or permanent basis. It is important to recognize that endogenous and exogenous compounds (eg, drugs, toxins, hemoglobin) alone or in combination with inappropriate renal blood flow (RBF) can promote or exacerbate renal disease.

Functions of the kidneys

The functions of the kidneys are as follows: (1) regulation of water, electrolyte, and acid-base balance; (2) regulation of blood pressure; (3) metabolism of endogenous and exogenous compounds; (4) excretion of endogenous waste products; (5) excretion of exogenous chemicals (xenobiotics); and (6) endocrine functions.

Various endogenous organic compounds eliminated by the kidneys include urea, creatinine, uric acid, indoles, phenols, skatoles, amines, heme byproducts (eg, bilirubin, urobilinogen), hormones, enzymes, and vitamins. The list of exogenous compounds eliminated by the kidney is extensive. Creatinine and urea are the two most frequently nitrogenous compounds measured in blood.

E-mail address: toribio.1@osu.edu

0749-0739/07/$ - see front matter © 2007 Elsevier Inc. All rights reserved.
doi:10.1016/j.cveq.2007.09.006

Functional renal anatomy

Most of the equine urinary tract is located in the retroperitoneal space. The equine kidneys have smooth surfaces with a less distinct corticomedullary junction than other species. The right kidney is heavier ($\sim$650 g) than the left kidney, with a horseshoe shape; it is located below the last two to three ribs and first lumbar transverse process, embedded into the liver, and it is approximately 15 cm long for an average-sized horse. The left kidney is elongated ($\sim$18 cm long, $\sim$600 g), more caudal than the right kidney, and can be palpated rectally. In newborn foals, each kidney weights around 170 g. The ratio of the kidneys to the body weight in equids is around 1:300.

The equine renal parenchyma is subdivided into 40 to 60 pyramids (cone-shaped arrangement of the renal tubules in the medulla) assembled in four rows, and at the tip of each pyramid is the papilla that projects into the renal pelvis and consists of large collecting ducts (ducts of Bellini). The equine renal papilla is sensitive to nonsteroidal anti-inflammatory drugs (NSAIDs) toxicity (papillary necrosis), in particular to phenylbutazone. This phenomenon seems to be the result of blood flow disruption and direct cell injury [1,2].

The renal pelvis represents a dilation of the ureter. The renal pelvis and proximal ureters have tubular glands and goblet cells that produce a mucous secretion that gives a viscous consistency to the normal equine urine. The ureters are 6 to 8 mm in diameter and 70 cm in length, with the last 5 cm traveling within the wall of the bladder. This last ureteral segment functions as a valve against vesicoureteral reflux during bladder distention, and it is important to reduce ascending infections. The equine bladder lies within the pelvis, except when it is filled or in certain bladder diseases (eg, sabulous cystitis), when it moves over the pelvic rim. Up to 4 L of urine can be in the bladder before the micturition reflex is triggered. In foals, the bladder is attached to the umbilical structures and it has an elongated form. As the foal gets older, these structures become the middle ligament (urachus) and the round ligaments (umbilical arteries). In addition, the bladder is held within the pelvis by the lateral ligaments. The urethra is 3 to 4 cm in the mare, whereas it is up to 90 cm in male horses.

Nephron

The functional unit of the kidney is the nephron. The nephron consists of a glomerulus, a proximal convoluted tubule, a loop of Henle with descending and ascending limbs, a distal convoluted tubule, a connecting tubule, and cortical and medullary collecting ducts. There are two types of nephrons: cortical and juxtamedullary nephrons. Cortical or superficial nephrons have short loops of Henle that extend a short way into the medulla, whereas juxtamedullary nephrons have their glomeruli located in the cortex, just above the corticomedullary junction, and have long loops of Henle that descend deep into the medulla (Fig. 1). There are variations among species in the cortical/juxtamedullary nephron ratio; however, this information is

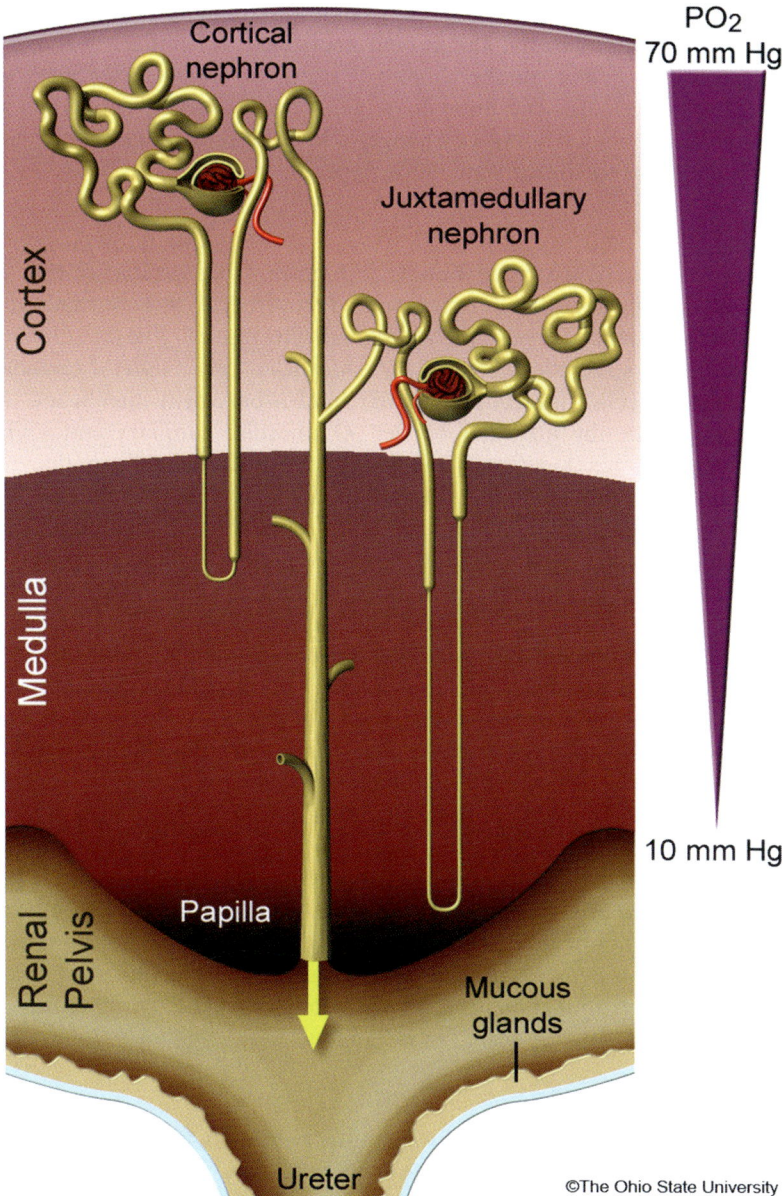

Fig. 1. Schematic representation of the nephron. There are two types of nephrons: cortical nephrons that have short loops of Henle and juxtamedullary nephrons with long loops of Henle. Mucous glands in the renal pelvis provide the viscous consistency of equine urine. (*Courtesy of* The Ohio State University, Columbus, OH; with permission.)

lacking in the horse. Each equine kidney has approximately 10 million nephrons [3,4]. Morphologically, the equine nephrons are similar to those of other species, and their number does not seem to increase after birth [3]. Renal disease decreases the number of nephrons; however, depending on the severity of damage, adaptive changes allow the remaining nephrons to increase their size to compensate (supernephrons).

Glomerulus

The glomerulus is a twisted bundle of high-pressure capillaries that receives blood from the afferent arteriole and, together with Bowman's capsule, forms the renal corpuscle (Malpighian corpuscle). The components of the glomerulus include the capillary endothelial cells, visceral epithelial cells, mesangial cells, intercellular matrix, and a basement membrane. All these layers make the filtration barrier. Glomerular capillary endothelial cells have large pores (fenestrae), and the visceral epithelial cells (podocytes) contain foot-like processes that extend to the basement membrane. The spaces between the foot processes are the slit pores (filtration slits), wherein final plasma filtration occurs. Endothelial cells, podocytes, and slit pores are covered with negative charges (eg, sialic acid, heparin sulfate) that repel the passage of large negatively charged molecules (proteins). The basement membrane's high content of proteoglycans also prevents the filtration of plasma proteins. Mesangial cells are not part of the filtration barrier but provide structural support to the glomerulus. Mesangial cells are contractile in response to local and systemic factors, secrete paracrine factors (prostaglandins), and therefore also affect the filtration rate.

Functions of the nephron include (1) ultrafiltration of plasma by the glomerulus; (2) reabsorption of water, solutes, and vitamins; (3) regulation of blood volume and pressure; (4) regulation of electrolytes and acid-base balance; (5) secretion of endogenous and exogenous compounds; (6) synthesis of endocrine, paracrine, and autocrine factors; (7) metabolic functions; and (8) excretion of urine. The processes performed by the nephron to create urine are (1) filtration of plasma by the glomerulus, (2) reabsorption of water and solutes, and (3) secretion of solutes.

Clinical implications

Knowing the basic anatomy of the equine kidneys is important, because congenital (renal dysplasia) and acquired disorders (eg, chronic renal failure, urolithiasis) alter the normal renal architecture. Diagnosing these conditions has therapeutic and prognostic implications. Please see the articles by Zellmer and Chaney elsewhere in this issue.

Innervation

Renal autonomic innervation is extensive. Sympathetic innervation is from the aorticorenal and celiacomesenteric ganglia, which contribute to the renal plexus, whereas parasympathetic innervation is from the vagus nerve. Renal innervation seems to be primarily sympathetic.

The main functions of renal autonomic innervation are (1) to control blood flow by regulating vascular resistance; (2) to control tubular cell function; (3) to activate the juxtaglomerular cells (renin secretion); and (4) to set the sensitivity of the tubuloglomerular feedback (TGF). Adrenergic stimulation increases RBF and diuresis. This is evident in horses with the administration of α_2-adrenergic agonists, such as xylazine and detomidine; however, the diuretic effects of these drugs seem to be mainly from adrenergic inhibition of vasopressin release (baroreceptor-mediated) and inhibition of vasopressin-mediated water reabsorption in the collecting ducts [5–7] rather than from glucosuria, as has been proposed [8]. Dopaminergic fibers increase RBF to the outer medulla and diuresis [9].

The ureters receive sympathetic and parasympathetic innervation from the celiac ganglion and pelvic nerve, respectively. The equine ureter has a dense adrenergic innervation [10,11]. α_1-Adrenergic stimulation increases ureter contractile activity, whereas β_2-adrenergic stimulation induces relaxation [11,12].

The bladder receives autonomic innervation from the hypogastric and pelvic nerves. For sympathetic innervation, preganglionic fibers from lumbar segments L1 to L4 synapse in the caudal mesenteric ganglia, from which adrenergic postganglionic fibers are carried to the bladder and the proximal urethra by the hypogastric nerve. In horses, β_2-adrenergic receptors are distributed throughout the bladder to induce detrusor muscle relaxation, which allows filling [10], whereas α_1-adrenoreceptors and, to a lesser extent, α_2-adrenoreceptors are distributed in the internal urethral sphincter to induce contraction and continence [13]. Parasympathetic cholinergic innervation is provided by the pelvic nerve, which carries postganglionic fibers from the sacral segments of the spinal cord. Stimulation of the pelvic nerve results in contraction of the detrusor muscle, relaxation of the internal urethral smooth muscle sphincter, and urination. Thus, bladder contraction is primarily a cholinergic process, which is important to understand clinically for the appropriate management of urinary incontinence (see the article by Schott elsewhere in this issue). Complete denervation of the bladder is unlikely to occur in the horse because there are nerve fibers that originate from ganglion cell bodies within the equine bladder wall [13]. The bladder receives somatic innervation from the pudendal nerve (S1–S2) to the external urethral sphincter and trigone, and it is critical in the tonic voluntary control of continence.

At least three areas of the central nervous system (CNS) control urination: (1) the cerebral cortex, (2) the brain stem micturition center (pons), and (3) the sacral micturition center. The micturition reflex center is mainly located in the first sacral segments of the spinal cord (parasympathetic contraction control). The pons is the major relay center between the cortex and the bladder. The pontine micturition center coordinates bladder contraction with sphincter relaxation (synergy). The cerebral cortex inhibits the pontine center and, indirectly, the sacral micturition center. Bladder stretching stimulates the pons and the cortex. In turn, the cortex removes inhibition to the pons → sacral stimulation → bladder contraction and sphincter relaxation → urination. Thus, micturition is a well-coordinated autonomic and conscious process in which cholinergic activation associated with sympathetic and pudendal inhibition results in urination.

Clinical implications

Several conditions are associated with bladder denervation, including trauma, spinal cord disease (eg, infectious, parasites, immune-mediated, compression, degeneration), peripheral neuropathies (eg, trauma, immune-mediated, toxic), and bladder disease (cystitis). Prolonged bladder distention may result in areflexia from lack of smooth muscle contractile activity (adynamic bladder disease). Reflex dyssynergia, a process in which detrusor contraction is not followed by urethral relaxation, is not a clearly defined condition in the horse. Understanding urinary tract innervation is important in the therapeutic management of urinary incontinence (see the article by Schott elsewhere in this issue).

Renal blood supply

Under resting conditions, the equine kidneys receive approximately 20% of the cardiac output [14,15]. Blood supply to the kidneys is provided by the renal arteries, which arise from the abdominal aorta and enter the kidney at the hilus, whereas the renal veins drain into the caudal vena cava. Each renal artery gives rise to lobar, interlobar, and arcuate arteries that branch into the cortex and lead to interlobular arteries, which give rise to the afferent arterioles and the glomerular capillaries (Fig. 2). The efferent arteriole from the glomerulus converges to a second capillary network around the renal tubules (peritubular capillaries) that descends into the medulla (see Fig. 2). The descending arterioles and peritubular capillaries, together with the larger ascending venules, are clustered together to form the vasa recta, which recovers water and solutes and provides the countercurrent mechanism required for urine concentration and to prevent the loss of electrolytes. Within the medulla, renal tubules and vasa recta are disposed in a hairpin pattern that maximizes urine concentration by countercurrent exchange [16]. Thus, the kidney has two capillary beds (glomerular and peritubular) that are arranged in series and have different functions. The high hydrostatic pressure at the glomerular capillaries induces fluid filtration, whereas the low hydrostatic pressure at the peritubular capillaries allows fluid and electrolyte reabsorption. These capillary networks are closely regulated by various autonomic, paracrine, autocrine, and endocrine mechanisms.

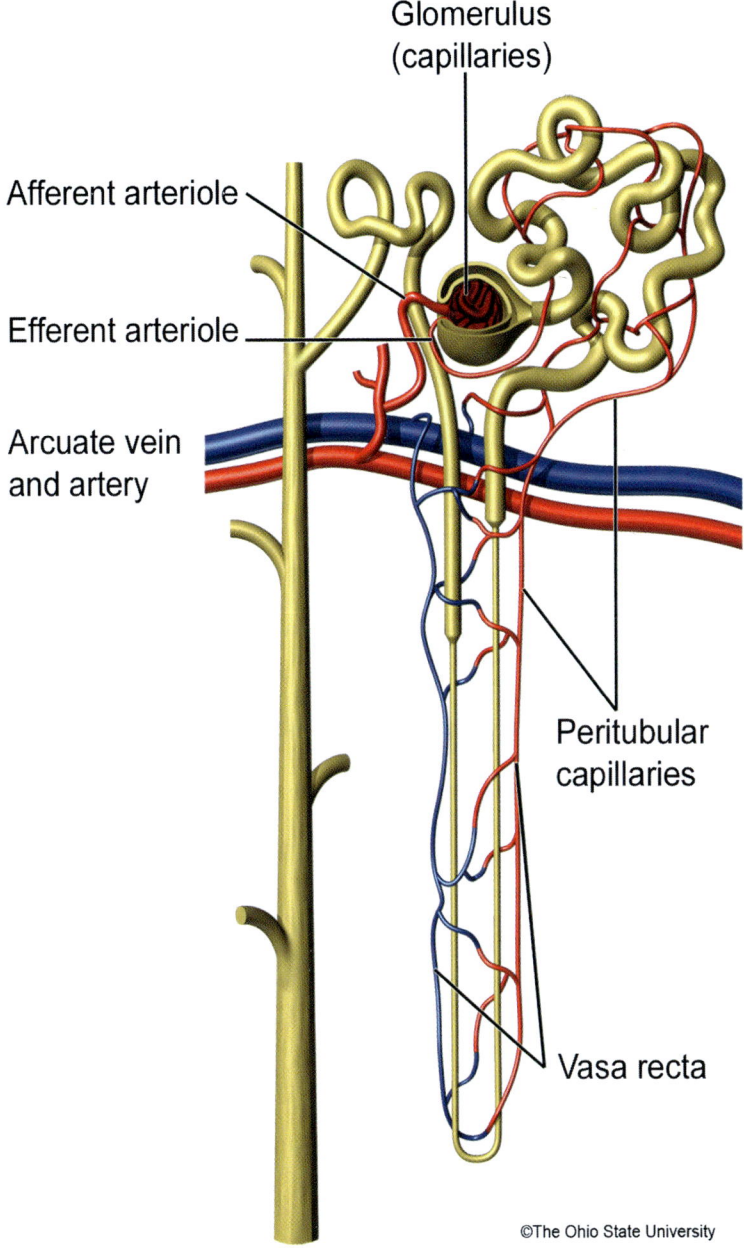

Glomerulus
(capillaries)

Afferent arteriole

Efferent arteriole

Arcuate vein
and artery

Peritubular
capillaries

Vasa recta

©The Ohio State University

Fig. 2. Representation of the renal blood supply. Renal arteries from the abdominal aorta give rise to lobar, interlobar, arcuate, and interlobular arteries. Interlobular arteries branch into afferent arterioles and glomerular capillaries. A second pericapillary network arises from the efferent arteriole. The descending arterioles, peritubular capillaries, and venules form the vasa recta that recover water and solutes and provide the countercurrent mechanism for urine concentration. (*Courtesy of* The Ohio State University, Columbus, OH; with permission.)

Renal blood flow

The kidneys are responsible for the fine regulation of body water, acid-base, and electrolyte balance. These functions are the result of RBF, glomerular filtration, tubular reabsorption, secretion, and diffusion and the effect of the renin-angiotensin-aldosterone system (RAAS). RBF determines the glomerular filtration rate (GFR) and the rate of energy-consuming processes, such as tubular reabsorption [17]. Thus, precise metabolic control of renal function requires accurate control of RBF (mainly by controlling the afferent arterioles).

The kidneys are second to the heart in regard to oxygen consumption, and relative to other organs and tissues, the kidneys have the highest blood flow; however, the renal oxygen extraction rate is low. The equine kidneys receive 15% to 20% of the cardiac output [14,15], which translates to 500 to 700 mL/min per 100 g of renal tissue, or 7 to 10 L/min of RBF for an average horse [14]. Based on several methods used to assess RBF in horses (eg, radionuclides, p-aminohippurate, microspheres, Doppler flow), RBF ranges from 10 to 25 mL/kg/min [4,14,15].

Despite the high RBF, the kidneys are susceptible to hypoxic injury as the result of a physiologic "redistribution" of blood flow and the low oxygen extraction rate [18]. Most of the RBF ($\sim$80%) is distributed to the renal cortex to improve glomerular filtration and proximal solute reabsorption, whereas less than 20% of the blood flow reaches the medulla by means of the vasa recta of the efferent arterioles to preserve osmotic gradients and enhance urinary concentration [4,16].

The diffusion of oxygen from arterial to venous vasa recta leaves the outer medulla deficient in oxygen. The medullary thick ascending limb of Henle generates the osmotic gradient for the active reabsorption of Na^+ by a process that requires large amounts of oxygen. The activity of Na^+/K^+ ATPase is responsible for approximately 70% of renal oxygen consumption [19]. Medullary hypoxia is a well-documented phenomenon in mammalian species, with partial pressures of oxygen in the medulla ranging from 10 to 20 mm Hg compared with 50 to 70 mm Hg in the cortex (see Figs. 1 and 2) [16]. Therefore, cells in the renal medulla live in a hostile environment characterized by wide variations of extracellular osmolality, low oxygen tensions, and abundant reactive oxygen species [20]. Juxtamedullary nephrons perform most of the concentration of urine and are the most susceptible to hypoxia.

Regulation of renal blood flow

To maintain proper renal blood supply, and therefore tubular function, there are autoregulatory mechanisms that control blood flow to the cortex, medulla, and individual nephrons. These include sympathetic activation, vasoconstrictors (eg, angiotensin II, norepinephrine, acetylcholine, endothelin-1), vasodilators (eg, prostaglandin E_2, adenosine, acetylcholine, bradykinin, dopamine, nitric oxide), and the TGF (Table 1). Compensatory mechanisms to protect the medulla from hypoxia include RBF redistribution from adenosine accumulation and increased production of prostaglandins and nitric oxide.

Juxtaglomerular apparatus and the tubuloglomerular feedback

The juxtaglomerular apparatus represents the structures formed by cells in the macula densa (junction of the thick ascending limb of the loop of Henle and the distal convoluted tubule), which are extraglomerular mesangial cells that fill the angle between afferent and efferent arterioles, smooth muscle, and renin-secreting cells (juxtaglomerular cells) in the afferent arteriole. This is the functional unit responsible for the TGF.

The TGF represents the mechanism by which the kidney regulates blood flow and GFR in individual nephrons, and therefore extracellular fluid and Na^+ balance. Because the fluid composition in the distal tubule is a function of the GFR, an increase in Na^+, K^+, and Cl^- indicates an elevated GFR. These electrolytes are sensed by the cells of the macula densa (by means of the $Na^+/K^+/2Cl^-$ cotransporter), which, in turn, increase extracellular adenosine concentrations that cause vasoconstriction of the afferent arteriole and decrease renin release [17]. In contrast, a decrease in Na^+ and Cl^- increases interstitial prostaglandin (I_2, E_2) production, which culminates in renin release (see section on RAAS). Dopamine, β-adrenergic agonists, and adrenomedullin also increase renin release. Dopamine agonists, such as fenoldopam, inhibit the TGF [21,22].

Renin-angiotensin-aldosterone system

The RAAS is an endocrine system that is essential in regulating blood pressure and extracellular fluid volume by controlling blood volume, cardiovascular function, and the renal excretion of water and electrolytes. Renin is an enzyme synthesized by the juxtaglomerular cells in response to renal artery hypotension, sympathetic innervation, and TGF (decreased Na^+ concentrations in the distal nephron stimulate renin release). Renin cleaves hepatic angiotensinogen to angiotensin I, which is converted to angiotensin

Table 1
Vasoactive factors affecting renal blood flow and glomerular filtration rate

Vasoconstrictors	Vasodilators
Epinephrine	Acetylcholine
Norepinephrine	Dopamine
Vasopressin	Prostaglandin E_2, I_2
Angiotensin II	Natriuretic peptides
Endothelin I	Nitric oxide
Thromboxanes	Bradykinin

II in the lungs by an angiotensin-converting enzyme. Angiotensin II causes systemic vasoconstriction and aldosterone and vasopressin release to increase renal Na^+ and water reabsorption. It also stimulates thirst, enhances sympathetic adrenergic function by facilitating norepinephrine release, inhibits vagal cardiac activity to produce tachycardia, and enhances Na^+ reabsorption in the renal tubules. Aldosterone increases tubular Na^+ reabsorption and K^+ secretion.

Vasoactive factors

Nitric oxide, a local vasodilator produced by cells of the macula densa, is important in medullary oxygenation and in reducing the metabolic rate of tubular cells. Adenosine is a vasodilator in the medulla, wherein it is released in response to hypoxia, and it is a potent vasoconstrictor for the afferent artery to reduce the GFR in response to increased tubular Na^+ and Cl^- [18,23]. ATP (adenosine precursor) seems to play a role similar to adenosine [23]. The role of vasodilatory prostaglandins on RBF is considered to be minimal under resting conditions but is important during renal vasoconstriction and hypoperfusion, particularly to the medulla and papilla. Dopamine increases RBF to the renal cortex and medulla; increases the GFR; and enhances tubular flow, natriuresis, and diuresis by inhibiting Na^+/K^+ ATPase [19]. Renal dopamine is primarily produced by the proximal tubular cells [24]. The intrarenal dopamine system seems to be a major regulator of Na^+ reabsorption [19]. All these properties make dopamine and dopaminergic agonists potential therapeutic options during equine renal hypoperfusion, in tubular obstruction, and to enhance natriuresis and diuresis [22,25]. Limited information on dopamine and equine renal function is available [19,25]. Angiotensin II increases the GFR by inducing efferent arteriole vasoconstriction and enhances Na^+ reabsorption (see section on RAAS). Endothelin-1 induces renal vasoconstriction and natriuresis (Table 1).

Clinical relevance

The kidneys have a high metabolic rate from the increased energy and oxygen demands of the tubular cells. Therefore, any process that decreases RBF, perfusion, or oxygenation can induce medullary hypoxic injury associated with tubular necrosis. Endogenous hemoproteins, such as hemoglobin and myoglobin, can cause severe renal vasoconstriction, acute tubular necrosis, and renal failure in the horse (see the article by Schumacher elsewhere in this issue). Hemoglobin, and to a lesser extent, myoglobin are the natural scavengers of nitric oxide, and their nephrotoxic effects are the result of vasoconstriction, tubular obstruction and necrosis, and Fe^{2+}-induced peroxidation. The use of NSAIDs to inhibit prostaglandin synthesis in horses, particularly phenylbutazone, predisposes to medullary ischemia, hypoxia, tubular cell necrosis, and papillary necrosis. This is exacerbated in horses with sepsis, endotoxemia, dehydration, poor renal perfusion, rhabdomyolysis, and hemolysis and with the use of nephrotoxic drugs (eg, aminoglycosides, polymyxin B, tetracyclines).

Glomerular filtration

Approximately 20% of the blood flowing through the kidneys is filtered by the glomeruli. Glomerular filtration is affected by the size, shape, and charge of the filtered particles. The glomerular capillary membrane is 100 to 400 times more permeable to ions than other capillary networks in the body. Most components of plasma are readily filtered across the filtration membrane, and their concentrations in the ultrafiltrate are similar to those in plasma. Molecules of less than 7 kilodaltons (kDa) are freely filtered, but in those greater than that, size, charge, and shape become more important. Proteins with molecular weights less than 60 kDa (eg, peptide hormones, enzymes, α_2-microglobulin) pass the filtration membrane to some extent. Negatively charged proteins (glycoproteins), regardless of size, have low filtration rates. Proteins with molecular weights around 65 kDa, such as albumin (69 kDa) and antithrombin III (60 kDa), are not found or are found in low concentrations in urine. Thus, the glomerular ultrafiltrate is a protein-free filtrate of plasma that contains water, electrolytes, and other solutes. Ionization is also important in the elimination of drugs bound to proteins; any change in pH that decreases protein binding increases drug elimination. Divalent cations bound to such proteins as calcium and magnesium are not filtered by the glomerulus, but ionized calcium (Ca^{2+}) and magnesium (Mg^{2+}) are freely filtered. Antimicrobials, such as aminoglycosides, fluoroquinolones, tetracyclines, imipenem, and sulfonamides, are eliminated by glomerular filtration and reach high urinary concentrations. Imipenem is combined with cilastin (inhibitor of renal dehydropeptidase) to decrease imipenem hydrolysis to nephrotoxic metabolites.

Clinical relevance

Understanding glomerular filtration is clinically relevant, because small-sized pigment proteins, such as hemoglobin and myoglobin (17 kDa), pass easily through the glomerulus and are nephrotoxic in horses (pigment-associated nephropathy; see the article by Schumacher elsewhere in this issue). In addition, glomerular disease can result in a protein-losing nephropathy that may lead to systemic signs (eg, edema, procoagulant state). Any renal condition that decreases glomerular filtration (eg, glomerulonephritis, dehydration, endotoxemia) results in azotemia (nitrogenous waste compounds in circulation) and in the systemic accumulation of drugs eliminated by filtration.

Renal tubular function

The movement of fluids, electrolytes, and endogenous and exogenous compounds in the renal tubules occurs by means of secretion, diffusion, and reabsorption. These processes are paracellular and transcellular; passive and active; voltage and concentration dependent; and regulated by humoral factors, electrolytes, extracellular volume, and the autonomic nervous system. Low-molecular-weight solutes that are essential for cell function and are filtered by the glomerulus (eg, glucose, amino acids) are effectively reabsorbed by the renal tubules and do not appear in urine (Figs. 3 and 4).

Water

Approximately 60% to 70% of water and solute (sodium chloride [NaCl]) reabsorption takes place in the proximal tubules by an isotonic (isosmotic), passive, paracellular process. As the ultrafiltrate moves through the loop of Henle and deeper into the medulla, it becomes hypertonic, because water in this segment of the nephron is reabsorbed in a higher proportion than solutes. Additional water reabsorption occurs in the collecting ducts mediated by vasopressin and aquaporin channels.

Sodium

Sodium transport across the renal tubules is paracellular and transcellular. Most Na^+ (60%–70%) is reabsorbed in the proximal tubes by isosmotic paracellular transport. Transcellular transport occurs by an Na^+/H^+ antiporter that facilitates bicarbonate ($HCO3^-$) reabsorption (proximal tubules), an Na^+/P_i cotransporter (proximal tubules) that facilitates phosphate (P_i) reabsorption, an $Na^+/K^+/2Cl^-$ cotransporter that facilitates Ca^{2+} and Mg^{2+} reabsorption (loop of Henle), an Na^+/Cl^- cotransporter (distal tubules), and an Na^+/K^+ ATPase (at the basolateral site of all tubular cells). Na^+ transport systems also facilitate glucose and amino acid reabsorption. The Na^+/K^+ ATPase generates the energy-dependent gradient for Na^+ reabsorption throughout the nephron, and it is responsible for roughly 70% of renal oxygen consumption [19]. Aldosterone (RAAS) increases Na^+ reabsorption by increasing the number and activity of Na^+/K^+ ATPases, whereas atrial natriuretic peptide (ANP) increases Na^+ excretion by inhibiting renin synthesis and release. Angiotensin II increases Na^+ resorption in the proximal tubules. Thus, in the proximal tubules, Na^+ reabsorption occurs with glucose, amino acids, P_i, and $HCO3^-$.

Glucose and amino acids

The transport of glucose in the proximal tubules is transcellular and associated with Na^+ transport. Because this is a carrier-mediated process, it is saturable and has a threshold that is a function of the amount glucose in plasma and the ultrafiltrate. The plasma threshold for glucose (plasma glucose concentrations at which glucose appears in urine) is estimated to be 150 to 200 mg/dL [4]. Amino acids are also transported in the proximal tubules by a process coupled with Na^+ transport. The threshold for amino acids is high (99% reabsorption).

Potassium

Potassium is reabsorbed in the proximal tubules by paracellular and transcellular processes. Potassium reabsorption in the proximal tubules and loop of Henle is closely associated with Na^+ reabsorption; however, in the distal tubules, K^+ is secreted, particularly under the influence of aldosterone. Metabolic alkalosis increases the urine secretion of K^+, whereas the opposite occurs with acidosis. Because the kidney is important in K^+ excretion, renal pathologic findings are often associated with hyperkalemia.

Bicarbonate

Approximately 80% of the filtered $HCO3^-$ is reabsorbed in the proximal tubules by a process that is linked to H^+ secretion and Na^+ reabsorption. Carbon dioxide (CO_2) diffuses from the lumen into the cytoplasm, where CO_2 + water (H_2O) $\rightarrow$ carbonic anhydrase $\rightarrow$ H_2CO_3 $\rightarrow$ HCO_3^- + H^+. Subsequently, HCO_3^- is extruded at the basolateral site by an HCO_3^-/Cl^- exchanger and an Na^+/HCO_3^- cotransporter (see Fig. 4), whereas H^+ is secreted back into the lumen in exchange for Na^+. This process is important not only for Na^+ and HCO_3^- reabsorption but for acid secretion (see Fig. 4). An inability to reabsorb HCO_3^- may result in type 2 (proximal) renal tubular acidosis (RTA), which is characterized by hyperchloremia and increased urine excretion of HCO_3^- and K^+, without azotemia [26,27]. The Fanconi syndrome, in which proximal tubular dysfunction results in type 2 RTA and decreased reabsorption of amino acids, glucose, and P_i, has not been clearly documented in the horse [28]; however, type 2 RTA has been described in horses [26,29,30]. Acetazolamide, an inhibitor of carbonic anhydrase, is effectively used in the management of horses with hyperkalemic periodic paralysis [31].

Acid secretion

Acid secretion occurs in all segments of the nephron. Active H^+ secretion by an $H^+/ATPase$ occurs in the intercalated cells of the distal and collecting tubules and is linked to HCO_3^- and K^+ reabsorption. A failure to secrete H^+ may result in type 1 (classic, distal) RTA, which is associated with hypokalemia and increased urinary excretion of K^+ and HCO_3^- [26,27]. The hypokalemia results from a lack of exchange between K^+ and H^+ that leads to excessive K^+ excretion and H^+ retention. Thus, type 2 RTA results from excessive base excretion, whereas type 1 results from acid retention. As with

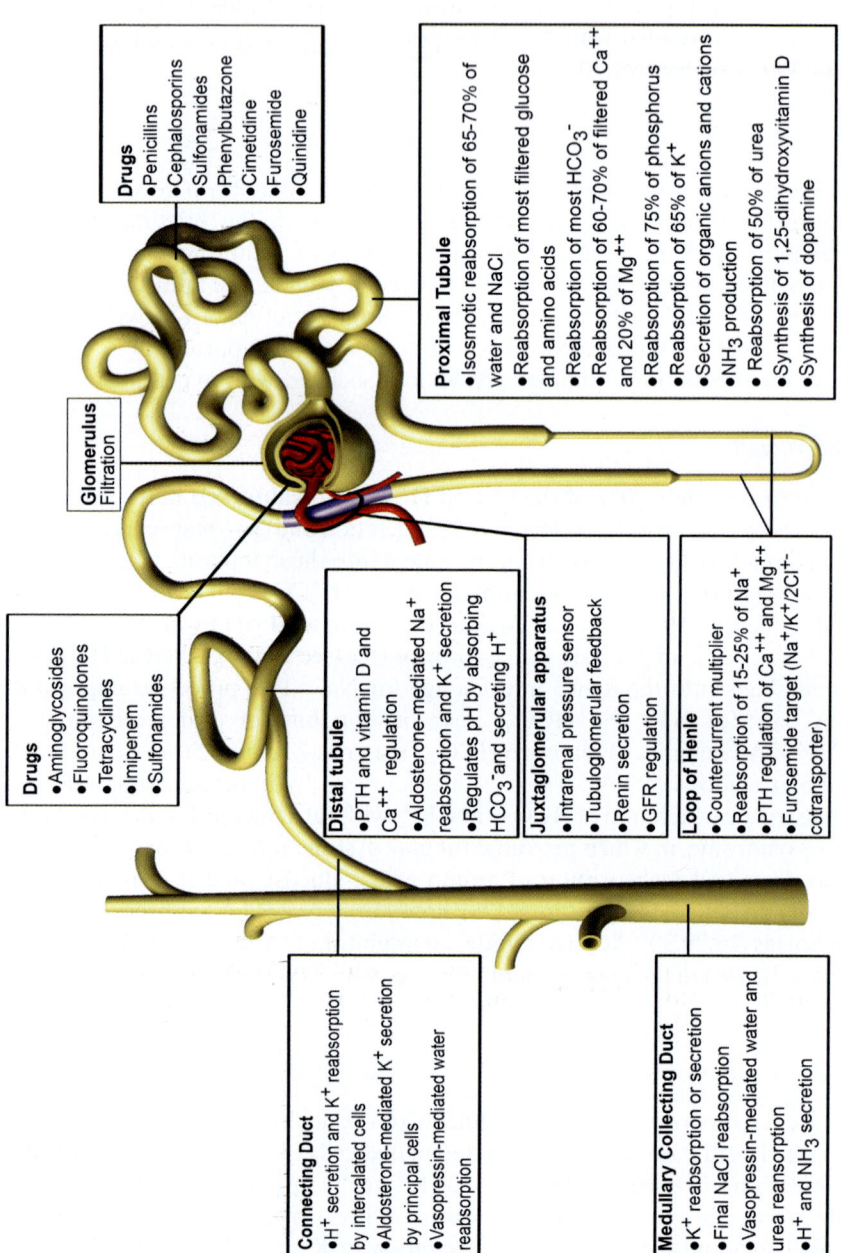

Drugs
- Penicillins
- Cephalosporins
- Sulfonamides
- Phenylbutazone
- Cimetidine
- Furosemide
- Quinidine

Proximal Tubule
- Isosmotic reabsorption of 65–70% of water and NaCl
- Reabsorption of most filtered glucose and amino acids
- Reabsorption of most HCO_3^-
- Reabsorption of 60–70% of filtered Ca^{++} and 20% of Mg^{++}
- Reabsorption of 75% of phosphorus
- Reabsorption of 65% of K^+
- Secretion of organic anions and cations
- NH_3 production
- Reabsorption of 50% of urea
- Synthesis of 1,25-dihydroxyvitamin D
- Synthesis of dopamine

Glomerulus
Filtration

Drugs
- Aminoglycosides
- Fluoroquinolones
- Tetracyclines
- Imipenem
- Sulfonamides

Distal tubule
- PTH and vitamin D and Ca^{++} regulation
- Aldosterone-mediated Na^+ reabsorption and K^+ secretion
- Regulates pH by absorbing HCO_3^- and secreting H^+

Juxtaglomerular apparatus
- Intrarenal pressure sensor
- Tubuloglomerular feedback
- Renin secretion
- GFR regulation

Loop of Henle
- Countercurrent multiplier
- Reabsorption of 15–25% of Na^+
- PTH regulation of Ca^{++} and Mg^{++}
- Furosemide target ($Na^+/K^+/2Cl^-$-cotransporter)

Connecting Duct
- H^+ secretion and K^+ reabsorption by intercalated cells
- Aldosterone-mediated K^+ secretion by principal cells
- Vasopressin-mediated water reabsorption

Medullary Collecting Duct
- K^+ reabsorption or secretion
- Final NaCl reabsorption
- Vasopressin-mediated water and urea reabsorption
- H^+ and NH_3 secretion

type 2 RTA, type 1 RTA has also been reported in horses [26,27,32]. The reader is referred to the article by Staempfli elsewhere in this issue for additional information on RTA. Diets with a low dietary cation-anion difference (acid diets) decrease urine pH and increase the excretion of calcium, magnesium, and P_i in various species, including the horse [33].

Phosphate

The kidney is the major regulator of serum P_i concentrations [34]. The proximal convoluted tubules reabsorb 7% to 80% of the filtered P_i and a small percentage in the distal segments of the nephron [34]. Phosphate transport is transcellular, unidirectional, and mediated by an apical Na^+/P_i cotransporter whose activity depends on the basolateral Na^+/K^+ ATPase [34–36]. Parathyroid hormone (PTH) and 1,25-dihydroxyvitamin D (calcitriol) are the main hormonal regulators of P_i excretion [37]. PTH inhibits and calcitriol increases P_i reabsorption in the proximal tubules. The urinary excretion of P_i is low in horses [35,36,38]. Hyperphosphatemia is a frequent finding in acute renal failure, whereas hypophosphatemia is common in chronic renal failure.

Calcium and magnesium

As for other electrolytes, the kidney is responsible for the fine regulation of extracellular Ca^{2+} and Mg^{2+}. Approximately 60% to 70% of Ca^{2+} and 20% of Mg^{2+} are reabsorbed in the proximal tubules by a paracellular process that requires water diffusion [36,37,39–41]. Most Mg^{2+} (50%–70%) and some Ca^{2+} (20%) reabsorption occurs in the thick ascending loop of Henle by the paracellular route and is driven by the positive voltage gradient generated by the $Na^+/K^+/2Cl^-$ cotransporter (see Fig. 4) [36]. The reabsorption of Ca^{2+} and Mg^{2+} in this segment of the nephron is controlled by PTH [36,37]. Fine regulation of these cations occurs in the distal nephron by means of transcellular mechanisms that are controlled by various hormones (eg, PTH, vitamin D, insulin, vasopressin, estrogen) [42–44]. The urinary excretion of Ca^{2+} and Mg^{2+} is higher in horses than in other species (Table 2). The high excretion of Ca^{2+} is the result of poorly regulated intestinal absorption of Ca^{2+} associated with efficient renal elimination. Thus, horses with chronic renal disease often develop hypercalcemia that is the result of Ca^{2+} retention and not from hyperparathyroidism as in small animals and human beings.

◄ ──

Fig. 3. Functions of the nephron. The nephron or functional unit of the kidney is active in physiologic processes, such as electrolyte, water, and acid-base balance; in the regulation of blood pressure; and in the excretion of various endogenous and exogenous compounds. (*Courtesy of* The Ohio State University, Columbus, OH; with permission.)

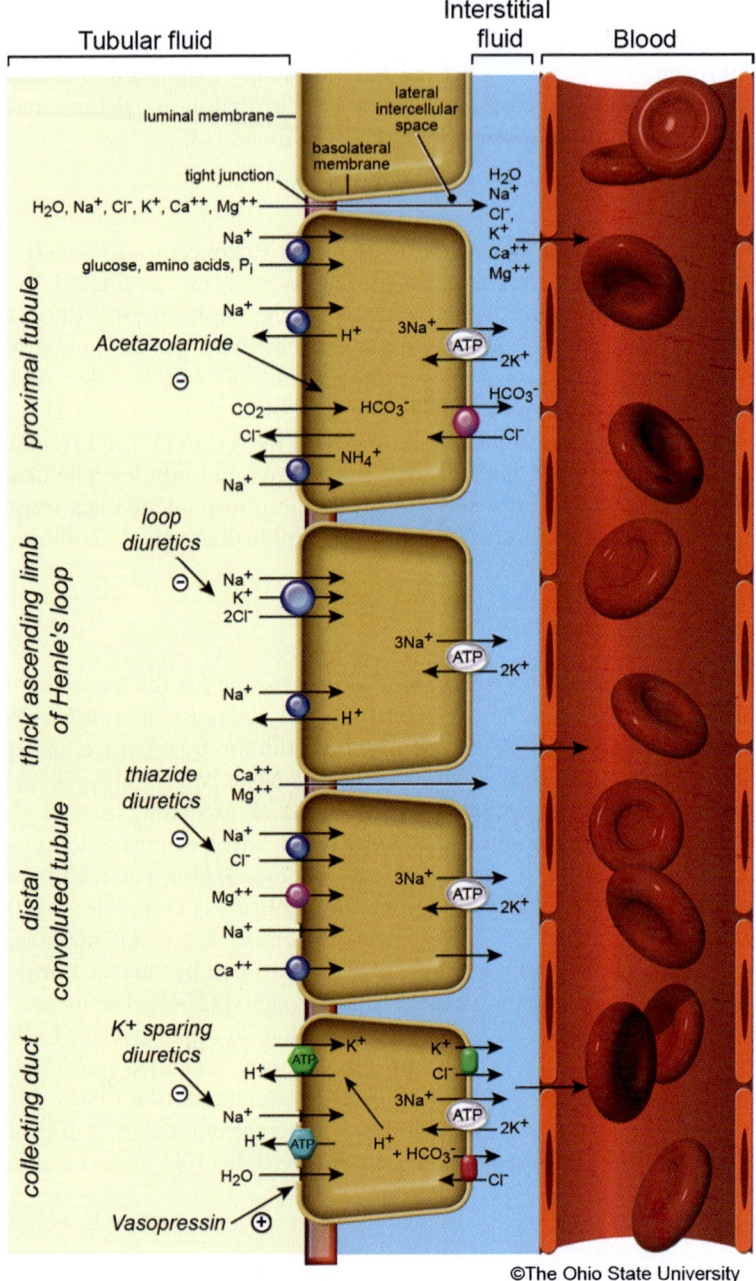

Fig. 4. Sites of solute, electrolyte, and acid-base regulation by the renal tubular cells. (*Courtesy of* The Ohio State University, Columbus, OH; with permission.)

Table 2
Indices of renal function in adult horses and foals

Variable	Adult	Foal
Serum BUN (mg/dL)	12–25	4–15
Serum creatinine (mg/dL)	0.8–2.2	0.7–1.2
F sodium (%)	0.01–1.0	0.01–0.2
F chloride (%)	0.01–1.0	0.01–0.4
F potassium (%)	20.0–80.0	10.0–30.0
F calcium (%)	3.0–10.0	2.0–6.0
F phosphorus (%)	0.0–0.5	0.5–5.0
F magnesium (%)	10–35	5.0–10.0
Urine specific gravity	>1.020	<1.008
Urine osmolality (mOsm/kg)	700–1500	<250
Urine pH	7.0–9.0	5.5–7.0
Urine production (mL/kg/h)	0.7–1.5	4.0–8.0

Abbreviation: F, fractional clearance of electrolyte in foals of less than 30 days of age.
Data from [4,33,35,36,38,49,52,58–66]; and the Veterinary Clinical Laboratory of The Ohio State University.

Organic anions and cations

Endogenous and exogenous anions eliminated by tubular secretion include cyclic adenosine monophosphate (cAMP), cyclic guanosine monophosphate (cGMP), prostaglandins, bile acids, hippurates, oxalate, urate, hormone metabolites (eg, estriol, estradiol, estrone), β-lactam antibiotics (eg, penicillin, ampicillin, cephalosporins), sulfonamides, probenecid, salicylates, digoxin, diuretics (eg, furosemide, ethacrynic acid, bumetanide, acetazolamide, thiazides), phenylbutazone, ascorbate, and folic acid [45]. Endogenous and exogenous cations eliminated by tubular secretion include choline, creatinine, dopamine, epinephrine, histamine, serotonin, cimetidine, ranitidine, procainamide, atropine, morphine, quinidine, and trimethoprim [45–48]. These compounds are primarily secreted by the proximal tubules, although some secretion also occurs in other segments of the nephron [45–48]. Quinidine and trimethoprim, drugs of frequent use in equine practice, decrease the tubular secretion of some drugs (eg, digoxin), increasing their potential toxicity [47]. Fluoroquinolones are excreted by glomerular filtration and tubular secretion, thus reaching high urinary concentrations. Aminoglycosides are excreted mainly by glomerular filtration (see the article by Schmitz elsewhere in this issue).

Clinical relevance

Any disease that interferes with proximal tubular cell function can result in Na^+ and HCO_3^- loss and in acid and Cl^- retention (ie, metabolic acidosis, RTA). One important renal function is to eliminate K^+, and renal pathologic findings are often associated with K^+ retention and hyperkalemia. The kidneys are essential in Ca^{2+} homeostasis, and acute renal failure is frequently associated with hypercalciuria, hypocalcemia, and hyperphosphatemia. In contrast, in chronic renal disease, the decreased GFR is frequently associated with Ca^{2+} retention, hypercalcemia, and hypophosphatemia. Because the kidneys are essential for acid-base homeostasis, any renal disease can result in metabolic acidosis.

Diuretics

The $Na^+/K^+/2Cl^-$ cotransporter is inhibited by furosemide, the Na^+/Cl^- cotransporter is inhibited by thiazide diuretics, and triamterene and amiloride inhibit Na^+ channels located in the principal cells of the late distal tubules and collecting ducts. Acetazolamide inhibits carbonic anhydrase in the proximal tubules to decrease reabsorption of $HCO3^-$ and Na^+ and increase K^+ secretion in the distal nephron (HYPP management). Aldosterone stimulates Na^+/K^+ ATPase to increase Na^+ reabsorption and K^+ secretion, whereas spironolactone (rarely used in horses), a competitive antagonist of aldosterone, increases Na^+ excretion and decreases K^+ (K^+-sparing diuretic) and H^+ excretion in the late distal tubule and collecting duct.

Countercurrent system: urine concentration

The countercurrent system refers to the mechanisms by which high medullary interstitial osmolarity is maintained to give the kidneys the ability to concentrate urine. The system consists of the loop of Henle and the vasa recta. The loop of Henle creates the medullary hyperosmolarity required for urine concentration (countercurrent multiplier), whereas the vasa recta allow the recirculation of solutes in the medulla (countercurrent exchanger).

Solutes diffuse out from the capillaries going to the cortex to capillaries descending into the medulla, whereas the opposite occurs with water. Thus, the countercurrent exchange of solutes between ascending and descending vasa recta minimizes the medullary "wash-out" of interstitial solutes (relevant to horses with polyuria/polydipsia) (see the article by MacKenzie elsewhere in this issue). NaCl and urea are the main medullary osmoles, with urea being the main osmole in urine.

Approximately 20% of Na^+ and Cl^- is reabsorbed in the loop of Henle. The descending loop of Henle is permeable to water and urea but is less permeable to Na^+ and Cl^-. Interstitial urea and Na^+ are responsible for water reabsorption in the descending limb. As the loop travels deeply into the medulla, the tubular fluid becomes more hyperosmolar (1200 mOsm/kg). In the ascending limb of the loop of Henle, Na^+ and Cl^- are transported by the $Na^+/K^+/2Cl^-$ cotransporter (K^+ is recycled back to the lumen) into the interstitial space, with a minimal amount of water being reabsorbed, thus creating a hyperosmotic medullary gradient that drives water reabsorption. As a result, the remaining hyposmotic tubular fluid is delivered to the distal tubules. This is known as the single effect, which is responsible for gradually increasing the interstitial osmolality from the renal cortex to the medulla and papilla.

As the hyposmotic tubular fluid moves through the distal tubules, it becomes isosmotic from water reabsorption. Vasopressin enhances water re-absorption in the collecting ducts. In the medullary collecting ducts, the tu-bular fluid loses more water to the hyperosmolar interstitium to be excreted, finally, as hyperosmolar concentrated urine.

Deep in the medulla and in the papilla, the single effect is repeated in fluid already submitted to the single effect (multiplication) to create a countercur-rent mechanism.

Clinical implications

Any condition that increases tubular flow and interferes with electrolyte re-absorption (eg, polyuria/polydipsia, psychogenic polydipsia) may result in medullary wash-out and decreased ability to concentrate urine (see the article by MacKenzie elsewhere in this issue). In general, horses with chronic renal failure lose the ability to dilute or concentrate urine and produce isosthenuric urine. In the hypoperfused/ischemic kidney, there is a decline in the GFR that leads to Na^+ retention and low urine production (eg, oliguric acute renal fail-ure, prerenal azotemia). If tubular damage is severe, the ability to reabsorb Na^+ and concentrate urine is lost, leading to nonoliguric or polyuric acute re-nal failure (see the article by Geor in this issue for additional information).

Assessment of renal function

Several methods are used in equine practice to evaluate renal function, including serum blood urea nitrogen (BUN), creatinine, and electrolyte con-centrations; indirect assessments of the GFR; urinary excretion of electro-lytes; fractional clearances; enzymuria; proteinuria; urine-concentrating capacity (specific gravity); and evaluation of the urine sediment. Even though these methods are valuable, the clinician should also be aware of their limitations.

Blood urea nitrogen

Urea is synthesized in the liver by the urea cycle enzymes from two am-monium ions that are produced during the catabolism of amino acids and nucleic acids. Ammonia (nonionic ammonium) is toxic to tissues, particu-larly to the CNS, whereas urea is less toxic. Because the liver is the site for urea synthesis, hepatic disease results in less urea production and lower circulating BUN concentrations. Most BUN ($>90\%$) is eliminated by the kidneys. Gastrointestinal excretion of urea is minimal because of bacterial degradation back to ammonia and enterohepatic circulation. BUN excre-tion also occurs in sweat and other body excretions. BUN is highly water soluble and equilibrates faster than creatinine between the intravascular and interstitial compartments.

Although BUN is a small molecule that is freely filtered at the glomerulus, it is a poor marker of the GFR because it can easily diffuse in and out of the renal tubules; its reabsorption is variable and linked to water and NaCl reabsorption. In the normal kidney, 40% to 70% of the BUN diffuses out into the interstitial space and back into systemic circulation. Therefore, BUN clearance underestimates the GFR (see the section on GFR). Unlike carnivores and omnivores, in which protein-rich diets increase BUN concentrations, diet has a minimal effect on BUN concentrations in the horse. In healthy newborn foals, BUN concentrations can be elevated in first days of life [49]. BUN concentrations are determined by various chemical and enzymatic methods, and results are reported in mg/dL (1 mg/dL = 0.357 mmol/L).

Creatinine

Serum creatinine is used in veterinary medicine as an indicator of the GFR, and thus to estimate renal function. Creatinine is the nonenzymatic byproduct of creatine P_i (phosphocreatine) in skeletal muscle. It is produced at a constant rate that is a function of muscle mass and body weight. Large horses and horses with a large muscle mass (eg, quarter horses, draft horses) tend to have higher creatinine concentrations, whereas horses with debilitating conditions tend to have low creatinine concentrations. Unlike carnivores, in which protein-rich diets affect creatinine concentrations, diet has no effect on serum creatinine in the horse and creatinine concentration is a direct function of muscle mass and renal function (GFR). Creatinine does not bind plasma proteins; it is filtered by the glomerulus, and, unlike other species, creatinine tubular reabsorption and secretion are minimal in the horse [50]. There is no enterohepatic circulation of creatinine, and gastrointestinal excretion may be important only during renal disease. Creatinine equilibration across the extracellular compartment is slower than that for BUN (4.0 versus 1.5 hours).

Serum creatinine concentrations of 3.0 to 5.0 mg/dL can be measured in healthy newborn foals [49]; as a general rule, they should decrease by 50% every day. After the first few days of life, creatinine concentrations in foals are lower than in adults as a result of decreased muscle mass and the higher GFR (see Table 2). Creatinine concentrations up to 30 mg/dL can be measured in premature foals and foals born to mares with placental insufficiency. These high creatinine values seem to result from placental dysfunction associated with the low diffusion of creatinine across the extracellular compartment (poor lipid solubility). Elevated creatinine concentrations do not cause uremia. Exercise can induce a mild increase in creatinine concentrations. Rhabdomyolysis is associated with increased creatinine concentrations, likely from muscle damage and myoglobin-mediated renal vasoconstriction and tubular necrosis. Creatinine concentrations can be increased in various pathologic conditions. Because creatinine equilibration across the extracellular compartments is slower than BUN, its concentrations in the peritoneal fluid are proportionally higher than BUN in patients that have uroabdomen.

Creatinine concentrations in body fluids are determined by a modified kinetic Jaffe reaction (alkaline picrate) and reported as mg/dL or μmol/L (1 mg/dL = 88.4 μmol/L). Hyperglycemia, hyperproteinemia, ascorbic acid, cephalosporins, ketones, and pyruvate produce Jaffe-like chromogens that overestimate serum creatinine concentrations, whereas hyperbilirubinemia falsely decreases creatinine concentrations. The problem of endogenous chromogens has been eliminated in most modern laboratories with the use of the modified Jaffe reaction.

Glomerular filtration rate

A substance can be excreted by glomerular filtration, tubular secretion, or both. Thus, the excretion of a substance is the result of glomerular and tubular functions. The GFR assesses glomerular function and blood flow, whereas the renal clearance evaluates tubular and glomerular functions:

$$\text{GFR} = \frac{U_x}{P_x} \times V$$

The GFR is considered the best test to assess kidney function and to determine the stage and progression of renal disease because it estimates the number of functional nephrons. The GFR is the rate at which a volume (milliliters) of fluid is filtered out of plasma per unit of mass (kilograms) and time (minutes) by the glomeruli. Therefore, the GFR is a function of the concentration of the substance in urine (U_x) and plasma (P_x) and the volume of urine (V) produced over time (minutes), and it is expressed as mL/kg/min.

In horses and ponies, the GFR ranges from 1.0 to 2.2 mL/kg/min, which is similar to other species [4,51–53]. This value is higher in foals (2.0–3.6 mL/kg/min) [54–56]. For an average-sized horse, this translates to a GFR per day of 1200 to 1400 L. Based on a urine production rate of 1.0 mL/kg/h, or 10 L/d, this value indicates that approximately 99% of the glomerular ultrafiltrate is reabsorbed by the renal tubules of the horse.

Factors that affect the GFR include those that influence RBF (blood volume, vascular resistance, autonomous neural input, and endocrine/paracrine/autocrine factors), osmolality, oncotic pressure, number and size of functional nephrons, glomerular disease, tubular disease, drugs, and toxins. The GFR can be measured using the inulin clearance method, iohexol, radiopharmaceuticals (eg, ^{125}I-iothalamate, ^{99m}Tc-diethylenetriaminepentaacetic acid [DTPA]), and endogenous products (creatinine).

Renal clearance

Renal tubular function can be assessed by the urinary excretion and clearance rates. The excretion rate is the amount of electrolyte eliminated over a period of time (mEq/min). The clearance rate of a substance or electrolyte (Cl_x) is the volume of plasma (milliliters) that contains the amount of the substance excreted in urine per unit of time (minutes) [57]. It is the amount of plasma that needs to be filtered to account for the amount of the substance present in urine every minute. As with the GFR, the clearance is a direct function of the concentration of the substance in urine (U_x) and plasma (P_x) and the volume of urine (V) collected over time (minutes), and it is expressed as mL/kg/min. Therefore, the clearance rate is similar to excretion rate, but it takes into account the GFR:

$$Cl_x = \frac{U_x}{P_x} \times V$$

The renal clearance of a substance (Cl_x) equals the GFR if the substance is excreted by glomerular filtration only. If the substance is filtered and secreted by the renal tubules, the Cl_x exceeds the GFR. If the substance is filtered and subsequently reabsorbed, renal clearance is less than the GFR. Therefore, the ideal filtration marker should be freely filtered by the glomerulus; should not be reabsorbed, secreted, synthesized, or metabolized by the renal tubular cells; and should be physiologically inert. Inulin is considered the ideal marker; however, using inulin in the equine clinical setting to assess the GFR is unrealistic and expensive. Endogenous substances, such as creatinine, that are primarily excreted by glomerular filtration can effectively be used to assess the GFR and renal function in the horse.

The creatinine clearance can be endogenous or exogenous. In the endogenous clearance, urine volume is measured over a period of time (6, 12, or 24 hours) and serum and urine creatinine concentrations are determined at the end of each interval [52]. The endogenous creatinine clearance (Cl_{cr}) in horses ranges from 1.0 to 2.5 mL/min/kg, which is similar to the GFR [51–53]. In the exogenous creatinine clearance, creatinine is injected and measurements are taken as before. The exogenous clearance is more accurate and reduces the effect of endogenous chromogens; however, its use is impractical and limited to research.

Fractional clearance of electrolytes

Because timed collection of urine is impractical, comparing the clearance of an electrolyte with that of a substance that reflects GFR (creatinine) is more realistic.

The fractional clearance of electrolytes (Fx) is calculated as [Ux/Sx]/[Ucr/Scr] × 100, where U is urine, S is serum, x is electrolyte concentration, and cr is creatinine concentration. Thus, the urinary fractional clearance is expressed as a percentage (%, fraction) of the clearance of creatinine. Some clinicians refer to this calculation as the fractional excretion. It is recommended that blood and urine samples be collected at the same time, although some flexibility is allowed, particularly if the animal is stable and not receiving fluid therapy or any treatment that interferes with urinary water and electrolyte excretion. Most studies comparing timed volumetric urine collections versus single-spot urine collections have found that a single measurement is adequate to assess renal function [58–61]. Samples should be collected preferably before feeding, exercise, or fluid therapy.

Because the function of the kidney is to retain most of the Na^+ and Cl^- in the ultrafiltrate, the fractional excretion of these electrolytes is less than 1% (see Table 2). The equine diet is rich in K^+, and its excretion is generally higher than 20%. The fractional of phosphorus is also low (<1%) and influenced by diet. Intestinal Ca^{2+} absorption is poorly regulated in the horse; therefore, its fractional excretion is high. The clinical value of evaluating urinary Ca^{2+} excretion in horses is unclear, because the normal range is wide and is affected by type of collection (voided versus catheter) and large quantities of calcium carbonate crystals are present in the urine sediment. Acute renal failure is associated with hypocalcemia and increased urine Ca^{2+} excretion, whereas chronic renal failure is associated with hypercalcemia from Ca^{2+} retention and decreased excretion (not from hyperparathyroidism as in other species) [35,36,38].

Although evaluating the urinary excretions of Ca^{2+} and phosphorus has been proposed to assess dietary intake, their value is limited because of the wide normal range and the poor intestinal regulation [37,62,67]. The excretion of Mg^{2+} is high in horses [36,38,58,59]. Early tubular damage is associated with increased excretion of Na^+, Cl^-, and phosphorus because their excretion under physiologic conditions is low. Increased excretion of Na^+ and Cl^- could also be the result of excessive intake. Caution should be taken in the interpretation of these results in the face of disease and treatments. Fluid therapy, furosemide, and hypercalcemia increase the excretion of electrolytes [36,68,69].

Proteinuria

Any condition that decreases the effective glomerular filtration barrier can result in proteinuria. A typical example is glomerulonephritis, although acute tubular necrosis and parenchymal inflammatory disease are also associated with proteinuria. Tamm-Horsfall protein (eg, mucoprotein, uromodulin) is a glycoprotein produced by the tubular cells of the thick ascending limb of the loop of Henle. Its concentration in urine is low, but it may be increased in renal inflammatory disease and forms the matrix for cellular and granular urinary casts [4].

Enzymuria

Because the kidney is a metabolically active organ, it is obvious that many of the enzymes present in the renal tubules can be detected in urine.

Any inflammatory, toxic, necrotic, ischemic, or degenerative condition that affects the tubular cells can increase the release of enzyme or enzyme-containing cells into urine. Thus, the measurement of tubular enzymes in equine urine has been advocated as a method to assess early renal disease [70–73]. Enzymes found in urine include small-molecular-weight enzymes filtered by the glomerulus but reabsorbed, tubular enzymes, and postrenal enzymes. Even though the number of enzymes detected in urine is high, few have diagnostic value in the horse. These include N-acetyl-β-D-glucosaminidase (NAG), lactate dehydrogenase (LDH), alkaline phosphatase (ALP), gamma-glutamyltransferase (GGT), and kallikrein [70–74]. The urinary activity of GGT and ALP seems to be greater in foals than in adults [49,70,72]. Except for GGT, measuring these enzymes on a routine basis is impractical. Although measuring GGT or the GGT/urine creatinine (GGT/Ucr) ratio may have some clinical use, the wide normal range has precluded its use by most clinicians. Further, horses with renal disease can have GGT/Ucr ratios that are in the normal range.

Clinical relevance

Serum creatinine is one of the most reliable tests to assess the GFR; however, because of the ability of the nephrons to compensate, it is estimated that greater than 75% of the renal functional mass must be lost before significant increases in creatinine are observed. Early-stage kidney disease can be present without major increases in serum creatinine concentrations. Because creatinine excretion is a direct function of RBF (and the GFR), any condition that decreases RBF (eg, hypovolemia, hypotension, dehydration) can increase serum creatinine concentrations (prerenal azotemia). If ischemia/hypoxia is severe or prolonged, prerenal azotemia can progress to acute renal failure (renal azotemia). The 50% creatinine prognostic rule in equine clinical practice implies that in horses with reversible renal damage and prerenal azotemia, serum creatinine should decrease between 40% and 60% in 24 hours if the animal receives proper hydration therapy. This information has been generated from clinical experience and has prognostic value.

Equine urine

Urine Formation = Glomerular Filtration

$$- \text{ (tubular reabsorption rate + secretion rate)}$$

Urine production in adult horses ranges from 1.0 to 2.0 mL/kg/h, whereas it ranges from 4.0 to 8.0 mL/kg/h in foals. This rate can increase or decrease depending on various conditions, including renal disease, water deprivation, dehydration, and psychogenic/neurogenic/nephrogenic polydipsia. The equine urine can have an osmolality (measured as the freezing point) of 1500 mOsm/kg and a specific gravity of greater than 1.025 (hypersthenuria), although healthy horses can produce dilute or concentrated urine. This value is five times the serum osmolality; thus, the equine kidney is extremely efficient in retaining water and Na^+ and, at the same time, eliminating waste osmoles like urea. Horses with chronic renal failure generally produce isosthenuric urine as the kidney loses the ability to dilute or concentrate urine. Normal equine urine color ranges from pale yellow to dark tan, and it is cloudy from the large quantities of calcium carbonate (and some calcium oxalate and P_i) and the presence of mucus. Equine urine may turn to a brown to red color after prolonged storage or air exposure from the presence of pyrocatechin (pyrocatechol), an oxidizing agent. Causes of urine discoloration should not be ignored, however. The equine urine is viscous from the presence of mucus produced by glands and goblet cells present in the renal pelvis and proximal ureters.

Like that of any herbivore, equine urine is alkaline, with a pH typically greater than 7.5 (range: 7.0–9.0). Diet, hydration, and various renal and bladder pathologic conditions affect urine pH. There should be no glucose in equine urine, unless there is renal disease or severe hyperglycemia or after α_2-agonist or glucocorticoid administration [8,75,76]. A positive result for blood should be interpreted with caution when using reagent strips because it may be the result of hemoglobin, myoglobin, or red blood cells or can be spurious in extremely alkaline urine. Protein concentration in equine urine is low (<100 mg/dL); however, reagent strips can yield false-positive results in alkaline samples. Expressing the protein/creatinine ratio is more practical because it eliminates timed collections. Proteinuria may be present in renal disease, urinary tract infections, and after exercise. GGT is an enzyme present in the brush border of the tubular cells, and urinary values greater than normal suggest tubular damage. The GGT/urine creatinine (GGT/Ucr) ratio is used by some clinicians to assess renal function.

Foal urine is clear, hyposthenuric (specific gravity <1.008, <250 mOsm/ kg), and acidic (pH 5.0–7.0), with more calcium oxalate crystals than in adults [49]. One study reported higher urine protein concentrations and GGT activity in foals than in adults [49], whereas other did not [60]. Urine specific gravity and osmolality can be elevated in healthy foals in the first day of life [49].

The equine urine sediment should be evaluated within 1 hour of collection or should be kept refrigerated until analysis (<24 hours). Because of the presence of large quantities of calcium salts in equine urine, some samples may require the addition of few drops of 10% acetic acid or hydrogen chloride (1/10 volume of 6 N HCl) to dissolve crystals for proper sediment evaluation. Casts are molds of tubular proteins (Tamm-Horsfall protein) that may contain systemic proteins, epithelial cells, cellular debris, erythrocytes, or leukocytes. Casts dissolve rapidly in the presence of alkaline urine, and there should be no casts in normal equine urine. The presence of erythrocytes depends on the method of collection, but there should be less than five red blood cells per high-power field in voided urine. The number of leukocytes should be less than five per high-power field.

Endocrine functions

Erythropoietin (EPO) is a glycoprotein synthesized by endothelial cells in the peritubular capillaries of the kidney in response to oxygen demands. EPO binds to its receptors on erythroid progenitors in the bone marrow to promote cell proliferation and maturation of erythrocytes [77].

Renin is an enzyme synthesized by the juxtaglomerular cells in response to renal artery hypotension, sympathetic innervation, and the TGF (described previously). Angiotensin II causes systemic vasoconstriction and aldosterone and vasopressin release to increase renal Na^+ and water reabsorption. It also stimulates thirst, facilitates norepinephrine release, and inhibits vagal cardiac activity to produce tachycardia and increase cardiac output.

Calcitriol (active vitamin D; 1,25-dihydroxyvitamin D) is synthesized from calcidiol (25-hydroxyvitamin D) by a 1α-hydroxylase enzyme located in the renal tubular cells, although the activity of this enzyme is low in the equine kidney (R.E. Toribio, unpublished data, 2007). Vitamin D synthesis is regulated by PTH, Ca^{2+} and P_i concentrations. Calcitriol stimulates intestinal absorption and renal reabsorption of Ca^{2+} and P_i, and it is important for bone mineralization and remodeling.

Clinical implications

Any renal disease associated with parenchymal damage (eg, chronic renal failure, interstitial disease) can result in nonregenerative anemia. Anemia can be exacerbated with the loss of vitamins that are reabsorbed by the tubules (folate, vitamin B_{12}). The use of human recombinant EPO (rhEPO) in horses has been associated with the production of anti-equine EPO antibodies and red blood cell aplasia [78].

References

[1] Khan KN, Paulson SK, Verburg KM, et al. Pharmacology of cyclooxygenase-2 inhibition in the kidney. Kidney Int 2002;61:1210–9.
[2] Sabatini S. Pathophysiologic mechanisms in analgesic-induced papillary necrosis. Am J Kidney Dis 1996;28:S34–8.
[3] Beech DJ, Sibbons PD, Rossdale PD, et al. Organogenesis of lung and kidney in thoroughbreds and ponies. Equine Vet J 2001;33:438–45.
[4] Schott HC. Disorders of the urinary system. In: Reed SM, Bayly WM, Sellon DC, editors. Equine internal medicine. St. Louis (MO): Saunders; 2004. p. 1169–294.
[5] Junaid A, Cui L, Penner SB, et al. Regulation of aquaporin-2 expression by the alpha(2)-adrenoceptor agonist clonidine in the rat. J Pharmacol Exp Ther 1999;291:920–3.
[6] Gellai M, Edwards RM. Mechanism of alpha 2-adrenoceptor agonist-induced diuresis. Am J Physiol 1988;255:F317–23.

[7] Xu H, Aibiki M, Seki K, et al. Effects of dexmedetomidine, an alpha2-adrenoceptor agonist, on renal sympathetic nerve activity, blood pressure, heart rate and central venous pressure in urethane-anesthetized rabbits. J Auton Nerv Syst 1998;71:48–54.

[8] Trim CM, Hanson RR. Effects of xylazine on renal function and plasma glucose in ponies. Vet Rec 1986;118:65–7.

[9] Chapman BJ, Horn NM, Robertson MJ. Renal blood-flow changes during renal nerve stimulation in rats treated with alpha-adrenergic and dopaminergic blockers. J Physiol 1982;325: 67–77.

[10] Labadia A, Rivera L, Costa G, et al. Influence of the autonomic nervous system in the horse urinary bladder. Res Vet Sci 1988;44:282–5.

[11] Prieto D, Hernandez M, Rivera L, et al. Catecholaminergic innervation of the equine ureter. Res Vet Sci 1993;54:312–8.

[12] Labadia A, Rivera L, Costa G, et al. Alpha- and beta-adrenergic receptors in the horse ureter. Rev Esp Fisiol 1987;43:421–5.

[13] Prieto D, Benedito S, Rivera L, et al. Autonomic innervation of the equine urinary bladder. Anat Histol Embryol 1990;19:276–87.

[14] Manohar M. Blood flow to the respiratory and limb muscles and to abdominal organs during maximal exertion in ponies. J Physiol 1986;377:25–35.

[15] Parks CM, Manohar M. Distribution of blood flow during moderate and strenuous exercise in ponies (Equus caballus). Am J Vet Res 1983;44:1861–6.

[16] Brezis M, Rosen S. Hypoxia of the renal medulla—its implications for disease. N Engl J Med 1995;332:647–55.

[17] Vallon V. Tubuloglomerular feedback and the control of glomerular filtration rate. News Physiol Sci 2003;18:169–74.

[18] O'Connor PM. Renal oxygen delivery: matching delivery to metabolic demand. Clin Exp Pharmacol Physiol 2006;33:961–7.

[19] Aperia AC. Intrarenal dopamine: a key signal in the interactive regulation of sodium metabolism. Annu Rev Physiol 2000;62:621–47.

[20] Neuhofer W, Beck FX. Survival in hostile environments: strategies of renal medullary cells. Physiology (Bethesda) 2006;21:171–80.

[21] Haberle DA, Konigbauer B. Inhibition of tubuloglomerular feedback by the D1 agonist fenoldopam in chronically salt-loaded rats. J Physiol 1991;441:23–34.

[22] Hollis AR, Ousey JC, Palmer L, et al. Effects of fenoldopam mesylate on systemic hemodynamics and indices of renal function in normotensive neonatal foals. J Vet Intern Med 2006; 20:595–600.

[23] Vallon V, Muhlbauer B, Osswald H. Adenosine and kidney function. Physiol Rev 2006;86: 901–40.

[24] Zhang MZ, Yao B, McKanna JA, et al. Cross talk between the intrarenal dopaminergic and cyclooxygenase-2 systems. Am J Physiol Renal Physiol 2005;288:F840–5.

[25] Trim CM, Moore JN, Clark ES. Renal effects of dopamine infusion in conscious horses. Equine Vet J Suppl 1989;7:124–8.

[26] Aleman MR, Kuesis B, Schott HC, et al. Renal tubular acidosis in horses (1980–1999). J Vet Intern Med 2001;15:136–43.

[27] Bayly WM. Renal tubular acidosis. In: Reed SM, Bayly WM, Sellon DC, editors. Equine internal medicine. St. Louis (MO): Saunders; 2004. p. 1283–6.

[28] Roberts MC, Seawright AA, Ng JC, et al. Some effects of chronic mercuric chloride intoxication on renal function in a horse. Vet Hum Toxicol 1982;24:415–20.

[29] MacLeay JM, Wilson JH. Type-II renal tubular acidosis and ventricular tachycardia in a horse. J Am Vet Med Assoc 1998;212:1597–9.

[30] Trotter GW, Miller D, Parks A, et al. Type II renal tubular acidosis in a mare. J Am Vet Med Assoc 1986;188:1050–1.

[31] Spier SJ, Carlson GP, Holliday TA, et al. Hyperkalemic periodic paralysis in horses. J Am Vet Med Assoc 1990;197:1009–17.

[32] Ziemer EL, Parker HR, Carlson GP, et al. Renal tubular acidosis in two horses: diagnostic studies. J Am Vet Med Assoc 1987;190:289–93.

[33] McKenzie EC, Valberg SJ, Godden SM, et al. Plasma and urine electrolyte and mineral concentrations in thoroughbred horses with recurrent exertional rhabdomyolysis after consumption of diets varying in cation-anion balance. Am J Vet Res 2002;63: 1053–60.

[34] Tenenhouse HS. Regulation of phosphorus homeostasis by the type IIa Na/phosphate cotransporter. Annu Rev Nutr 2005;25:197–214.

[35] Toribio RE, Kohn CW, Chew DJ, et al. Comparison of serum parathyroid hormone and ionized calcium and magnesium concentrations and fractional urinary clearance of calcium and phosphorus in healthy horses and horses with enterocolitis. Am J Vet Res 2001;62: 938–47.

[36] Toribio RE, Kohn CW, Rourke KM, et al. Effects of hypercalcemia on serum concentrations of magnesium, potassium, and phosphate and urinary excretion of electrolytes in horses. Am J Vet Res 2007;68:543–54.

[37] Toribio RE. Disorders of the endocrine system. In: Reed SM, Bayly WM, Sellon DC, editors. Equine internal medicine. St. Louis (MO): Saunders; 2004. p. 1295–379.

[38] Toribio RE, Kohn CW, Hardy J, et al. Alterations in serum parathyroid hormone and electrolyte concentrations and urinary excretion of electrolytes in horses with induced endotoxemia. J Vet Intern Med 2005;19:223–31.

[39] Friedman PA. Codependence of renal calcium and sodium transport. Annu Rev Physiol 1998;60:179–97.

[40] Friedman PA. Calcium transport in the kidney. Curr Opin Nephrol Hypertens 1999;8: 589–95.

[41] Edwards BR, Baer PG, Sutton RA, et al. Micropuncture study of diuretic effects on sodium and calcium reabsorption in the dog nephron. J Clin Invest 1973;52:2418–27.

[42] Brown EM, MacLeod RJ. Extracellular calcium sensing and extracellular calcium signaling. Physiol Rev 2001;81:239–97.

[43] Satoh J, Romero MF. Mg2+ transport in the kidney. Biometals 2002;15:285–95.

[44] Hoenderop JG, Bindels RJ. Epithelial Ca2+ and Mg2+ channels in health and disease. J Am Soc Nephrol 2005;16:15–26.

[45] Moller JV, Sheikh MI. Renal organic anion transport system: pharmacological, physiological, and biochemical aspects. Pharmacol Rev 1982;34:315–58.

[46] Inui KI, Masuda S, Saito H. Cellular and molecular aspects of drug transport in the kidney. Kidney Int 2000;58:944–58.

[47] Masereeuw R, Russel FG. Mechanisms and clinical implications of renal drug excretion. Drug Metab Rev 2001;33:299–351.

[48] Launay-Vacher V, Izzedine H, Karie S, et al. Renal tubular drug transporters. Nephron Physiol 2006;103:97–106.

[49] Edwards DJ, Brownlow MA, Hutchins DR. Indices of renal function: values in eight normal foals from birth to 56 days. Aust Vet J 1990;67:251–4.

[50] Finco DR, Groves C. Mechanism of renal excretion of creatinine by the pony. Am J Vet Res 1985;46:1625–8.

[51] Walsh DM, Royal HD. Evaluation of a single injection of 99mTc-labeled diethylenetriaminepentaacetic acid for measuring glomerular filtration rate in horses. Am J Vet Res 1992;53: 776–80.

[52] Morris DD, Divers TJ, Whitlock RH. Renal clearance and fractional excretion of electrolytes over a 24-hour period in horses. Am J Vet Res 1984;45:2431–5.

[53] Matthews HK, Andrews FM, Daniel GB, et al. Comparison of standard and radionuclide methods for measurement of glomerular filtration rate and effective renal blood flow in female horses. Am J Vet Res 1992;53:1612–6.

[54] Gonda KC, Wilcke JR, Crisman MV, et al. Evaluation of iohexol clearance used to estimate glomerular filtration rate in clinically normal foals. Am J Vet Res 2003;64:1486–90.

[55] Brewer BD, Clement SF, Lotz WS, et al. A comparison of inulin, para-aminohippuric acid, and endogenous creatinine clearances as measures of renal function in neonatal foals. J Vet Intern Med 1990;4:301–5.

[56] Holdstock NB, Ousey JC, Rossdale PD. Glomerular filtration rate, effective renal plasma flow, blood pressure and pulse rate in the equine neonate during the first 10 days post partum. Equine Vet J 1998;30:335–43.

[57] DiBartola SP. Applied renal physiology. Fluid, electrolyte and acid-base disorders in small animal practice. Philadelphia: Elsevier Saunders; 2005. p. 26–44.

[58] McKenzie EC, Valberg SJ, Godden SM, et al. Comparison of volumetric urine collection versus single-sample urine collection in horses consuming diets varying in cation-anion balance. Am J Vet Res 2003;64:284–91.

[59] Stewart AJ, Hardy J, Kohn CW, et al. Validation of diagnostic tests for determination of magnesium status in horses with reduced magnesium intake. Am J Vet Res 2004;65:422–30.

[60] Brewer BD, Clement SF, Lotz WS, et al. Renal clearance, urinary excretion of endogenous substances, and urinary diagnostic indices in healthy neonatal foals. J Vet Intern Med 1991; 5:28–33.

[61] Kohn CW, Strasser SL. 24-Hour renal clearance and excretion of endogenous substances in the mare. Am J Vet Res 1986;47:1332–7.

[62] Caple IW, Bourke JM, Ellis PG. An examination of the calcium and phosphorus nutrition of thoroughbred racehorses. Aust Vet J 1982;58:132–5.

[63] Caple IW, Doake PA, Ellis PG. Assessment of the calcium and phosphorus nutrition in horses by analysis of urine. Aust Vet J 1982;58:125–31.

[64] Edwards DJ, Brownlow MA, Hutchins DR. Indices of renal function: reference values in normal horses. Aust Vet J 1989;66:60–3.

[65] Grossman BS, Brobst DF, Kramer JW, et al. Urinary indices for differentiation of prerenal azotemia and renal azotemia in horses. J Am Vet Med Assoc 1982;180:284–8.

[66] Rawlings CA, Bisgard GE. Renal clearance and excretion of endogenous substances in the small pony. Am J Vet Res 1975;36:45–8.

[67] Lane VM, Merritt AM. Reliability of single-sample phosphorus fractional excretion determination as a measure of daily phosphorus renal clearance in equids. Am J Vet Res 1983;44:500–2.

[68] Hinchcliff KW, Mitten LA. Furosemide, bumetanide, and ethacrynic acid. Vet Clin North Am Equine Pract 1993;9:511–22.

[69] McKeever KH. Effect of exercise on fluid balance and renal function in horses. Vet Clin North Am Equine Pract 1998;14:23–44.

[70] van der Harst MR, Bull S, Laffont CM, et al. Gentamicin nephrotoxicity—a comparison of in vitro findings with in vivo experiments in equines. Vet Res Commun 2005;29:247–61.

[71] Adams R, McClure JJ, Gossett KA, et al. Evaluation of a technique for measurement of gamma-glutamyltranspeptidase in equine urine. Am J Vet Res 1985;46:147–50.

[72] Brobst DF, Carroll RJ, Bayly WM. Urinary enzyme concentrations in healthy horses. Cornell Vet 1986;76:299–305.

[73] Bayly WM, Brobst DF, Elfers RS, et al. Serum and urinary biochemistry and enzyme changes in ponies with acute renal failure. Cornell Vet 1986;76:306–16.

[74] Giusti EP, Sampaio CA, Michelacci YM, et al. Horse urinary kallikrein, I. Complete purification and characterization. Biol Chem Hoppe Seyler 1988;369:387–96.

[75] Simon F, Laczay P, Mora Z, et al. Target animal safety test of a dexamethasone-prednisolone combination in horses. Dtsch Tierarztl Wochenschr 1990;97:339–40, 342.

[76] Thurmon JC, Steffey EP, Zinkl JG, et al. Xylazine causes transient dose-related hyperglycemia and increased urine volumes in mares. Am J Vet Res 1984;45:224–7.

[77] Lacombe C, Da Silva JL, Bruneval P, et al. Erythropoietin: sites of synthesis and regulation of secretion. Am J Kidney Dis 1991;18:14–9.

[78] Piercy RJ, Swardson CJ, Hinchcliff KW. Erythroid hypoplasia and anemia following administration of recombinant human erythropoietin to two horses. J Am Vet Med Assoc 1998; 212:244–7.

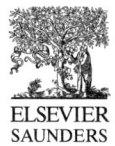
ELSEVIER
SAUNDERS

VETERINARY
CLINICS
Equine Practice

Vet Clin Equine 23 (2007) 563–575

Examination of the Urinary Tract in the Horse

M. Eilidh Wilson, BVMS

*Department of Large Animal Clinical Sciences, D-202 Veterinary Medical Center,
Michigan State University, East Lansing, MI 48824–1314, USA*

The urinary tract includes the kidneys, the ureters, the bladder, the urethra, and, in the male, the accessory glands. Pathologic conditions of the urinary tract may produce specific clinical signs, such as stranguria, but they are more than likely to be nonspecific clinical signs, such as lethargy and weight loss, which often occur with chronic renal disease in addition to countless other diseases. Further, clinical signs that may seem to be directly related to the urinary tract, such as polyuria, polydipsia, or red-stained urine, may be the result of other systemic diseases. Thus, before embarking on diagnostics, it is important to obtain a thorough history and physical examination.

History

A complete history should include signalment (age, breed, and gender), the role of the horse (pasture pet versus performance horse), the presenting complaint, the husbandry of the horse, and a history of previous problems and drug administration.

Important concerns that relate to the urinary tract should include how much the horse drinks. This may be difficult for an owner to determine, especially if automatic water machines are used or the horse is pastured. A normal horse should drink approximately 60 to 65 mL/kg/d, which equates to 30 to 32.5 L/d for a 500-kg horse. Unless there is an obvious reason for increased intake (eg, fluid losses in sweating or diarrhea), drinking in excess of this amount is polydipsia. Owners should be encouraged to monitor this closely over a 24-hour period. An effective way to do this is simply to confine the horse and offer a known volume of water. Because water

---

E-mail address: wilso716@cvm.msu.edu

doi:10.1016/j.cveq.2007.10.001

intake changes depending on the horse's diet, work level, and environmental temperature, it is best to repeat this experiment several times.

Urine output may be much harder for the owner to determine. Information regarding urine frequency and volume is important. Polyuria is the excessive excretion of urine resulting in excessive micturition. Pollakiuria describes excessive frequency of micturition, and dysuria is difficulty or pain in micturition. Incontinence is involuntary voiding of urine. It may be hard for an owner to differentiate between polyuria and pollakiuria. The distinction is important, however, because polyuria is more suggestive of a renal abnormality and pollakiuria, dysuria, and incontinence reflect a problem distal to the kidney.

A normal adult horse should produce urine at a rate between 5 and 15 L/day. Twenty-four–hour urine collection may be achieved with an indwelling Foley urinary catheter with a closed collection set. This is often not always practical, because not all animals tolerate this and there is risk for introduction of bacteria. Other methods have been described for noninvasive collection from geldings. A gallon container is modified (capped at the top and the base is removed and padded) and is secured to the ventral abdomen in front of the prepuce by suspending it from gauze roll that is wrapped around the lumbar back and then between the legs. The horse urinates into the container, which must be emptied regularly.

If hematuria is the complaint, further information with regard to timing within the urinary stream may aid your diagnosis. Blood at the beginning of the stream may indicate a urethral or accessory gland problem. Blood at the end or throughout the stream is more suggestive of the problem originating in the bladder or kidneys. In addition, does the hematuria occur with each urination? A common presenting complaint with urolithiasis is hematuria after exercise.

A history of any previous conditions may be relevant to urinary tract disease. Urolithiasis can occasionally cause signs of colic, and vague signs of lethargy or weight loss may occur with chronic renal failure (CRF). Any history of nephrotoxic medications is also essential.

Physical examination

In addition to a normal physical examination, other details should be sought. Uremia associated with CRF can cause excessive tartar, buccal, or tongue ulcerations and halitosis. Ventral edema may indicate a protein-losing nephropathy, and more obvious signs, such as alopecia and ulceration (urine scalding) of the perineum or hind legs, may indicate incontinence.

It is essential to perform rectal palpation when investigating the urinary tract. The bladder may be palpated just over the pelvic rim. The bladder should be evaluated for size (distention can be indicative of obstruction or neurogenic abnormality, thickening of the wall, intramural masses [tumors], and intraluminal masses [cystic calculi, clots, or sabulous material]).

The caudal pole of the left kidney can be palpated, and abnormalities in size and texture may be appreciated. Ureters are not normally appreciable on rectal examination; however, they may be prominent if they are distended, such as with obstructive uterolithiasis.

Laboratory data

Complete analysis of the urinary tract includes examination of blood (serum chemistry and hematology) and urine.

Evaluation of hematology and serum chemistry

Glomerular filtration is the first step of urine formation. In the average horse, the glomerular filtration rate (GFR) is 0.6 to 2.0 mL/kg/min, meaning 12,000 to 14,000 L of plasma is filtered per day in a 500-kg horse. To measure the filtration rate accurately, it is necessary to select a substance that is only filtered by the glomerulus and is not reabsorbed or secreted by the tubules. Inulin (a plant polysaccharide) is such a substance, which is used experimentally. Thus, the rate of clearance from the blood is the result of glomerular filtration only. Elevations in blood inulin are indicative of a reduction in GFR.

Clinically, creatinine and blood urea nitrogen (BUN) are useful indicators of GFR. Creatinine is a waste product formed in the muscle. Like inulin, it is freely filtered, and the excretion rate is essentially equal to its filtration (ie, concentrations are unaltered by the tubules). Again, like inulin, plasma creatinine concentrations vary inversely with GFR. Like creatinine, BUN, a byproduct of amino acid metabolism, is also a useful indicator of GFR but is less sensitive to changes in GFR than creatinine. This is because creatinine is produced at a relatively constant rate and is similarly presented to the kidneys at a constant rate.

This is not true of BUN, in which production may be altered. Increased production can follow gastrointestinal bleeding, and reductions may occur because of liver failure or a low-protein diet. BUN is also low in foals because of the high rates of protein synthesis.

Further, BUN excretion is not solely determined by filtration. Once in the tubules, approximately 40% to 50% of BUN is then reabsorbed into the surrounding interstitium, and this urea transport is enhanced during hypovolemic states. This can result in elevations in BUN that are not directly associated with or correspond to reductions in GFR.

Azotemia is a term that means an elevation in nonprotein nitrogenous proteins and clinically relates to increases in creatinine and BUN. This is a laboratory finding. *Uremia* ("urinary constituents within the blood"), conversely, is a term that relates to the clinical manifestations observed with renal failure, such as halitosis, dental plaque, oral ulceration, inappetence, and nausea. Azotemia develops consequent to a reduction in GFR and may be further characterized as prerenal, renal, or postrenal azotemia.

Prerenal azotemia occurs secondary to dehydration or hypovolemia, leading to reduced renal blood flow, and, generally, is not as great as that induced by intrinsic renal azotemia. Typically, with prerenal azotemia, the BUN may elevate to a greater extent than the creatinine.

The BUN/creatinine ratio is a calculation that was created to try to aid in differentiation of intrinsic renal azotemia from prerenal azotemia based on the proportional increases of BUN and creatinine. Dehydration results in increased tubular reabsorption of BUN, leading to a much greater elevation in BUN compared with creatinine, which is not associated with a reduction in GFR. Thus, in dogs, an elevated BUN/creatinine ratio may be suggestive of prerenal azotemia.

In the case of uroperitoneum (most commonly seen in foals with bladder rupture), the lipid-soluble structure of BUN promotes reabsorption through the peritoneum into the blood, resulting in much greater elevations in BUN compared with creatinine.

With an abrupt decrease in functional renal glomeruli (renal azotemia), the creatinine increases proportionately more than the BUN, resulting in a low BUN/creatinine ratio. In dogs a BUN/creatinine ratio may be helpful in characterizing the source of the azotemia, but there is such a wide variation in BUN and creatinine concentrations with all three causes of azotemia that it is not a reliable indicator [1]. In the horse, a BUN/creatinine ratio of less than 10:1 is expected with acute renal failure (ARF), and when the ratio exceeds 15:1, CRF is more likely.

Thus, the degree of azotemia cannot definitively characterize its cause. A specific gravity (SG) must be obtained for this, with an elevated SG (>1.035 indicating concentrated urine) being present during dehydration or hypovolemia (prerenal) and an abnormal SG suggesting renal damage.

The kidney has a large reserve, and when renal azotemia is detected, it indicates that approximately 75% of the nephrons are no longer functioning. Thus, monitoring elevations in creatinine and BUN is not sensitive to mild or moderate reductions in GFR. Once azotemia is detected, however, further elevations in BUN and creatinine are sensitive for continued loss of functional mass, with a doubling of creatinine or BUN indicative of a further 50% decline in the remaining functional nephrons.

Postrenal azotemia in the horse most commonly occurs secondary to bladder rupture (seen in neonates) and urethral obstruction (often secondary to urolithiasis, especially in male horses). In the case of a ruptured bladder, uroperitoneum develops. In foals, the most common location of the tear is the dorsal aspect of the bladder, and because of this location, many continue to posture and seem to urinate normally. Abdominal distention ultimately develops, however, as the abdomen continues to fill with urine.

Uroperitoneum is confirmed by analysis of the peritoneal fluid for creatinine. Detection of high levels of creatinine (twofold increase compared with venous values) is indicative of disruption of the urinary tract. It must be remembered that although the bladder is the most common area that is ruptured in foals, other areas may be damaged, such as the ureters or the urachus.

Protein-losing nephropathies resulting in hypoproteinemia seem to be less common in the horse than in companion animals. During glomerulonephritis, damage to the glomerular filtration barrier occurs, allowing larger molecules and charged molecules to pass into the ultrafiltrate. When the ability of the tubules to reabsorb proteins is overwhelmed, proteinuria develops. Primarily, albumin is lost, resulting in hypoalbuminemia.

Hypercalcemia and hypophosphatemia are often found with CRF, and hypocalcemia and hyperphosphatemia are more common with ARF. Hyperkalemia is commonly observed with ARF (especially oliguric or anuric renal failure) and also with urinary obstruction or, most commonly, in foals with uroperitoneum.

Hyponatremia is variably reported in renal disease, but hypochloremia is a consistent finding with polyuric renal failure [2].

Renal tubular acidosis (RTA) is characterized by altered renal tubular function and results in a hyperchloremic metabolic acidosis [3]. Blood gas analysis reveals a pH less than 7.23, with chloride concentrations as low as 106 to 121 mEq/L. Bicarbonate is also decreased at less than 13 mEq/L. The anion gap (AG) should be normal:

$$AG = \{(Na+) + (K+)\} - \{(Cl-) - (HCO_3)\}$$

with a reference range of 6 to 15 mEq/L. In a study of 16 horses affected by RTA, however, 4 affected horses had a slightly elevated AG attributable to other forms of intrinsic renal disease [3].

Analysis of globulins and white blood cell count may indicate an infectious process, such as pyelonephritis. Assessment of red blood cell count and muscle activity may provide further information when assessing red-colored urine (hematuria or hemoglobinuria).

Urinalysis

The color of urine should be noted. The color of normal urine is similar to that of cider. Adult equine urine is alkalotic and contains a lot of mucus and calcium carbonate crystals. This may be appreciated toward the end of urination, when the urine appears cloudier and there are more numerous crystals passed in the urine. Foal urine is acidic, and calcium oxalate crystals are more prevalent [4].

SG estimates the solute concentration of the urine. SG is defined as the weight of a solution compared with its equal volume of distilled water.

Plasma, which is approximately 0.8% to 1% heavier than [5] distilled water, has an SG of 1.008 to 1.010. SG is measured with a refractometer (things that alter it, such as hemoglobin), and thus can be easily assessed. This is only an estimate of concentration, however, and osmolality (defined as the number of particles per kilogram of water) is a more accurate determinant. Because SG is proportional to solute weight and number, the weight of large molecules, such as glucose or albumin, increases the SG by a larger amount than the osmolality increases with these particles. When glucosuria or proteinuria is present, an osmolality measurement should be obtained, because the SG will be much higher than the actual osmolality of the urine.

Urine concentration may be classified in one of three ways. The first is urine that is less concentrated than plasma, known as hyposthenuria (SG <1.008 and an osmolality of <269 mOsm/kg). Urine that is similar to plasma concentration (and glomerular filtrate) is termed *isosthenuria* (SG: 1.008–1.012 and an osmolality of 260–300 mOsm/kg). Urine that is more concentrated than plasma is called hypersthenuric (SG >1.012 and an osmolality >300 mOsm/kg). Normal adult horses produce concentrated (hypersthenuric) urine. Azotemia in conjunction with hypersthenuria (SG >1.035) is supportive of a prerenal cause, with the release of antidiuretic hormone (ADH) and resultant concentration of urine. Failure to concentrate the urine in the face of azotemia is supportive of renal disease.

Foals on a milk diet produce hyposthenuric urine because of the large fluid volume that is ingested and their large urine output (mean urine production of 148 ± 20 mL/kg/d compared with mean urine production of 14.7–25.1 mL/kg/d in the adult horse) [6,7]. Their BUN and creatinine also remain at subadult levels while this hyposthenuria is maintained [4]. They concentrate their urine in the face of dehydration or a change of diet, however.

Small solutes (eg, electrolytes) are freely filtered at the glomerulus (similar to creatinine). The tubules then alter the ultrafiltrate by reabsorbing or secreting solutes. The fractional clearance (FC; also referred to as fractional excretion) determines the clearance of a solute excreted in the urine and compares this with the clearance of creatinine and its excretion in the urine. If a solute were to be filtered at the glomerulus and pass through the tubules unaltered (eg, creatinine) it would be equal to creatinine (1.0). FC evaluates tubular function:

$$FCx = (U_x P_{Cr})/(U_{Cr} P_x) \times 100$$

where FCx is the fractional clearance of electrolyte X, U_X is the urine concentration of electrolyte X; P_{Cr} is the plasma concentration of creatinine; U_{Cr} is the urine concentration of creatinine, and P_X is the plasma concentration of electrolyte X.

FC is usually expressed as a percentage. In the normal horse, all solutes have an FC less than 1 (100%), because the body conserves solutes. The tubules resorb approximately 99% of sodium and chloride, producing fractional excretions of less than 1%. The FC of sodium may help to distinguish prerenal from renal azotemia. In dehydrated animals, the FC should be low, because the body tries to conserve sodium. In contrast, if there is a primary renal problem (tubular damage), the FC increases to greater than 1%.

Diet and intravenous crystalloid fluids may also increase the FC of sodium, however. In these cases, there is an increased sodium load in the plasma, which increases the filtered load, and the tubules try to excrete the excess.

The normal FC for potassium is higher (range: 15%–65%). Once again, a diet high in potassium increases the FC. With anorexia, the FC decreases as the body attempts to conserve the solute.

The FC of phosphorus may also be affected with diets that are high in phosphates or low in calcium. Elevations in FC for sodium and phosphorus may be an early indicator of renal tubular damage, however.

Calcium carbonate crystals are abundant within equine urine; thus, accurate assessment of FC requires that the bladder be completely emptied and that the urine be processed to dissolve all the crystals. Therefore, calcium should not be assessed on routine urinalysis.

The FC of foals has been investigated. The FC for sodium is similar to that for adults, but the FC is increased for potassium, phosphorus, and calcium [4].

Ideally, when measuring a serum sample, the sample should be obtained at a time similar to that when the urine sample is obtained.

γ-Glutamyltransferase (GGT) is a brush-border enzyme that has high concentrations on the proximal convoluted tubule. Increased GGT activity in the urine has been associated with tubular damage. GGT activity is assessed as a ratio with creatinine to reduce the variability that occurs with urine volume excreted by the kidneys.

It is recognized that a GGT/creatinine ratio greater than 25 IU/g is abnormal and does indicate tubular damage; however, clinically, these minor elevations seem to be subclinical. This is the downfall of this test. Elevations in the GGT/creatinine ratio are observed after routine treatment with nephrotoxic gentamicin. Thus, the high sensitivity of this test makes it hard to interpret these results [2].

Extremely large elevations (> 100 IU/g) may precede azotemia, however, and may have more clinical relevance. This test is not used commonly in practice because of its tendency to detect subclinical disease.

A transient and marked proteinuria is often detected in foals after colostrum ingestion (for the first 48 hours) [4]). Colostrum results in an increase in small proteins within the plasma, which are filtered in the glomerulus. The concentration of protein overwhelms tubular reabsorption, and proteinuria results.

Proteinuria may be detected on commercial dipsticks. Normal herbivore urine is alkalotic, however, and this can result in false-positive proteinuria results. Hemoglobin can also create false-positive results. More sensitive methods for detecting proteinuria include sulfosalicylic acid precipitation, the trichloroacetic acid method or Coomassie brilliant blue assay, or benzethonium chloride assay.

In the adult horse, the mean value for 24-hour urine protein excretion is 3.2 mg/kg, although a variation has been reported (3.6–22.3 mg/dL). Determination of the urinary protein–to–urinary creatinine (Up/UCr) ratio eliminates the necessity of 24-hour urine collection. Although a normal range has not been determined for the horse, a ratio greater than 1.0:1 is considered abnormal in the dog and is accepted as abnormal in horses also.

Glomerulonephritis causes a defect in the filtration barrier such that larger charged molecules, such as albumin, can pass from the blood into the ultrafiltrate. This results in proteinuria, and when it is severe enough, it causes hypoalbuminemia. Protein-losing nephropathy is not as common in the horse as in companion animals. Other causes for proteinuria include pyuria and bacteruria, and it also occurs after exercise. A sediment analysis should be performed when evaluating proteinuria. The presence of proteinuria accompanying active sediment is suggestive of an inflammatory renal disease or inflammatory disease of the lower urinary tract or genital tract.

Glucose is freely filtered by the glomerulus but ordinarily is reabsorbed by a glucose cotransporter in the proximal convoluted tubule. Glucosuria develops when the tubules are overwhelmed or damaged. The transport threshold for horses is approximately 150 mg/dL, which is lower than in dogs and cats. When glucosuria and hyperglycemia are present, it is suggestive of a systemic cause, such as equine metabolic syndrome, pituitary intermedia dysfunction, or elevated catecholamines or cortisol, which may be seen with corticosteroid therapy, intense exercise, pain, stress, or shock. It should also be noted that α_2-antagonists result in a transient glucosuria. When normoglycemia is present, glucosuria is indicative of proximal tubule dysfunction.

Ketones are rarely detected in equine urine. Unlike ruminants, horses rarely become ketotic.

Bilirubinemia indicates increased circulation of conjugated bilirubin. Hemolytic disease, hepatic disease, or posthepatic obstruction may all result in elevated bilirubin, and investigation to rule out these disorders should be pursued.

Urobilirubin is a breakdown product of bilirubin that is formed in the intestine. It is absorbed by the intestines but is not removed by the portal circulation and is ultimately excreted in the urine. Its presence only indicates a patent bile duct, and increases may be detected with hemolytic, hepatic, or posthepatic diseases. Neither the reagent strips nor assays can be used to detect negative urobilinogen.

Urinary sediment evaluation is important to evaluate the urinary tract thoroughly. In approximately 16% of dogs that have normal physical and chemical evaluation of urine, there are actually abnormal sediment findings (eg, pyuria, bacteruria, microscopic hematuria). This highlights the importance of sediment evaluation. The contents of urine are not stable. Cells and casts deteriorate, and crystals may dissolve or form; thus, urine should be analyzed within a few hours of collection. This is the most likely reason why urinary sediment evaluation is underutilized in equine medicine [8].

The method of collection should be considered because it can affect the analysis. Sediment is first examined on a low-power field (lpf) to look for casts. The presence of cells (red blood cells, white blood cells, and epithelial cells) are recorded per high-power field (hpf) [9].

Casts are cylindrically shaped molds that are formed within the kidney tubules and are composed of glycoprotein and cells. Some casts (especially hyaline casts) dissolve in alkaline urine; thus, sediment analysis should be performed promptly after collection if possible. Detection of casts indicates a tubular abnormality.

Pyuria is present when more than five white blood cells per hpf are seen. In dogs and cats, normal values are zero to eight white blood cells per hpf for a voided sample, zero to five per hpf for a catheterized sample, and zero to three per hpf for a cystocentesis, illustrating that the method of collection may affect the white blood cell count. Pyuria indicates inflammation or infection but does not localize the site unless white blood cell casts are viewed, which would indicate pyelonephritis.

Less than five red blood cells per hpf is normal (if the sample collection is atraumatic). Hematuria (> 5 red blood cells per hpf) can occur with trauma, urolithiasis, inflammation, infection, toxemia, neoplasia, or exercise. Similar to pyuria, it does not localize the source unless red blood cell casts are present.

Hematuria may be detected with reagent strips, where it is actually the heme that is detected. Heme may originate from hemoglobin or from myoglobin. Thus, a positive result on a reagent strip does not differentiate between intact erythrocytes in the urine, free hemoglobin (hemoglobinuria), or myoglobinuria.

Hematuria can occur from trauma, hemorrhage, urolithiasis, inflammation, or neoplasia, for example. Hemoglobinuria indicates intravascular hemolysis with subsequent filtration of the hemoglobin into the tubules. Myoglobinuria may occur after severe myopathies, such as trauma or rhabdomyolysis. Unfortunately, an assay to differentiate between hemoglobinuria and myoglobinuria is not commonly available, but a diagnosis can usually be reached by evaluating hematology and serum chemistries [10].

Bacteria maybe visualized, but the absence of bacteria does not exclude their presence. For this reason, a culture is required. Culture should only be performed if the sample is aseptically collected by means of catheterization or cystocentesis (which may be performed in foals), because a voided sample most likely has bacteria attributable to catheterization [9].

The water deprivation test is used to evaluate patients that have polydipsia and hyposthenuric polyuria when other causes for polyuria and polydipsia have been excluded. It is usually performed to determine if a horse has psychogenic polydipsia or diabetes insipidus.

The test is contraindicated in animals that are azotemic or dehydrated. In such cases, the hyposthenuria is likely caused by an intrinsic renal abnormality.

To perform the test, the bladder is catheterized and completely emptied. At this point, baseline data are collected (creatinine, BUN, hematocrit, plasma proteins, urine osmolality and SG, and body weight). Water is then withheld, and the body weight and urine SG are monitored every 4 to 6 hours. Normal horses respond appropriately and concentrate their urine. Producing urine with an SG of 1.025 indicates normal function and suggests psychogenic polydipsia. The test should be discontinued if more than 5% of the body weight is lost.

An inability to concentrate urine with a water deprivation test (provided there is no azotemia or clinical signs of dehydration) is suggestive of diabetes insipidus [11]. To determine if it is nephrogenic or central, exogenous ADH may be administered. Desmopressin acetate (DDAVP) can be safely used. In central diabetes insipidus, the SG should increase to greater than 1.020 within 2 to 7 hours of administration of desmopressin acetate. If no change is detected, nephrogenic diabetes insipidus can be diagnosed.

Bacteria may be visualized, but the absence of bacteria does not exclude their presence. For this reason, a culture is required. Culture should only be performed if the sample is aseptically collected by means of catheterization or cystocentesis (which may be performed in foals), because a voided sample most likely has bacteria attributable to catheterization.

Ultrasound

Ultrasound of the bladder is best performed with transrectal ultrasound using a 5- MHz probe. Normal urine is echogenic because of the presence of crystals and mucus. These contents should swirl on manipulation of the bladder. Focal wall thickening, wall defects, or masses may be visualized. Cystic calculi can be palpated on rectal examination; however, when using transrectal ultrasound, they appear as a hyperechoic line that casts an acoustic shadow. These are most commonly located at the bladder trigone. Stones lodged in the urethra may also be felt rectally and confirmed with ultrasound.

The kidneys may be visualized with transabdominal ultrasound using a 2.5- to 3-MHz probe in an adult horse. The left kidney is positioned medial to the spleen in the paralumbar area and may be difficult to visualize because of its deeper position. The right kidney is usually easier to image and is visualized just beneath the body wall through the dorsolateral aspect of the last two to three intercostal spaces.

The kidneys should be imaged in longitudinal and cross section. The normal size for adult equine kidneys is less than 15 cm long for the right kidney and less than 18 cm long for the left kidney.

The kidneys may be enlarged in ARF and small with CRF. The parenchyma should be assessed. A distinct cortex and medulla should be visible, although this is sometimes hard to assess in large or fat horses. The cortex is homogeneous in echogenicity, and the medulla is more hypoechoic. The renal pelvis is echogenic because of the presence of intrapelvic fat and fibrous tissue and appears as a longitudinal bright white echo that traverses through the middle of the kidney when viewing the longitudinal axis. Changes in size, shape, architecture, and echogenicity may all be detected.

Changes that may be observed with ARF include renal enlargement and perirenal edema. Usually, the kidneys appear less echogenic. CRF may reveal small irregular kidneys or increased echogenicity.

Cystic kidneys are detectable, because there is replacement of normal architecture with hypoechoic cysts. Nephrolithiasis or mineralization can be identified as a bright hyperechoic density that casts an acoustic shadow. Hydronephrosis is also detected as a dilated pelvis and renal calyces and is indicative of obstructive disease [12].

Congenital renal disease, such as renal cysts, or renal hypoplasia may be detected on ultrasound examination.

When a ruptured bladder and uroperitoneum are suspected, abdominal ultrasound usually indicates an increase in hypoechoic peritoneal fluid. If the urinary bladder is ruptured, a small flaccid bladder is detected and the defect in the bladder may often be located. If a tear in the ureter has occurred, the bladder appears normal but is surrounded by hypoechoic fluid. Analysis of the peritoneal fluid confirms uroperitoneum, and retrograde contrast studies or exploratory studies help to localize the defect.

Radiography can really only be used to evaluate foals or miniature horses. An intravenous pyelogram (IVP) may be performed to diagnosis such defects as nonfunctional kidneys, ectopic ureters, or hypoplastic kidneys.

Retrograde contrast studies may be performed to evaluate urethral or bladder defects. They provide little advantage over endoscopy, however.

Endoscopy of the urinary tract is easy to perform. A flexible videoendoscope can be used (<12 mm in diameter, 1 m long). This procedure should be performed aseptically. The patient is sedated, and the genitals are thoroughly cleaned. The bladder is first catheterized to remove any urine. The sterile endoscope is passed into the urethra in exactly the same way that the catheter was passed.

The endoscope should pass easily through the urethra. Minor trauma can often occur during passage. In geldings or stallions, particular attention should be paid to the urethra at the level of the ischial arch, because this is a common area for urethral rents or tears.

After entering the bladder, it will be necessary to insufflate with air to ensure that the entire bladder and mucosa can be visualized easily. The presence of cystic calculi, sabulous material, masses, and inflammation should be visible. The ureteral openings are visible at 10 and 2 o'clock positions at the trigone. Urine should drain from these openings in intermittent bursts (approximately once every minute). If no urine is produced, that kidney is not functional. Occasionally, when ureters are dilated, it is possible to enter and travel proximal toward the kidney. Dilated ureters are suggestive of congenital or, more commonly, obstructive disease. If the ureters are of normal diameter, a rigid catheter (number 8–10 French polypropylene catheter) can be passed to collect urine samples, which may help to localize renal hemorrhage or pyelonephritis. Unilateral renal hematuria can often be observed with the endoscope alone by observing the color of the urine as it enters the bladder.

Nuclear scintigraphy can be applied to access renal anatomy and function and is most necessary when individual renal function must be determined, such as before a nephrectomy.

Biopsies can easily be obtained through the biopsy channel. A renal biopsy provides a histologic diagnosis but should really only be considered when the information may change the treatment of the patient. It is relatively safe, although complications that can occur include perirenal hemorrhage, hematuria, and bowel perforation.

The patient should be sedated and restrained. The biopsy is ultrasound guided. The needle (Tru-Cut biopsy needle) is directed toward the parenchyma, and tissue is harvested.

References

[1] Finco DR, Duncan JR. Evaluation of blood urea nitrogen and serum creatinine concentrations as indicators of renal dysfunction: a study of 111 cases and a review of related literature. J Am Vet Med Assoc 1976;168(7):593–601.
[2] Carr AE. Examination of the urinary system. In: Robinson NE, editor. Current therapy on equine medicine. 5th edition. Philadelphia: Saunders; 2003. p. 819–24.
[3] Aleman MR, Kuesis B, Schott HC, et al. Renal tubular acidosis in horses (1980–1999). J Vet Intern Med 2001;15:136–43.
[4] Edwards DJ, Brownlow MA, Hutchins DR. Indices of renal function: values in eight normal foals from birth to 56 days. Aust Vet J 1990;67(7):251–4.
[5] Rose BD, Post TW. Meaning and application of urine chemistries. In: Rose BD, Post TW editors. Clinical physiology of acid-base and electrolyte disorders. 5th edition. New York: McGraw-Hill Medical Publishing Division; 2001. p. 405–15.
[6] Kohn CW, Strasser SL. 24-Hour renal clearance and excretion of endogenous substances in the mare. Am J Vet Res 1986;47(6):1332–7.
[7] Brewer BD, Clement SF, Lotz WS, et al. Renal clearance, urinary excretion of endogenous substances, and urinary diagnostic indices in healthy neonatal foals. J Vet Intern Med 1991; 5(1):28–33.
[8] Barlough JE, Osborne CA, Stevens JB. Canine and feline urinalysis: value of macroscopic and microscopic examinations. J Am Vet Med Assoc 1981;178(1):61–3.
[9] DiBartola SP. Renal disease: clinical approach and laboratory evaluation. In: Ettinger SJ, Feldman EC, editors. Textbook of veterinary internal medicine, volume 2. 6th edition. Missouri: Elsevier Saunders; 2005. p. 1716–30.

[10] Stockham SL, Scott MA. Urinary system. In: Stockham SL, Scott MA, editors. Fundamentals of veterinary clinical pathology. Ames (IA): Blackwell; 2002. p. 277–337.

[11] Schott HC 2nd, Bayly WM, Reed SM, et al. Nephrogenic diabetes insipidus in sibling colts. J Vet Intern Med 1993;7(2):68–72.

[12] Reef VB. Adult abdominal ultrasound. In: Reef VB, editor. Equine diagnostic ultrasound. Philadelphia: WB Saunders; 1998. p. 273–363.

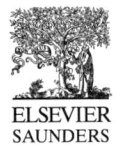

ELSEVIER
SAUNDERS

VETERINARY
CLINICS
Equine Practice

Vet Clin Equine 23 (2007) 577–591

Acute Renal Failure in Horses

Raymond J. Geor, BVSc, MVSc, PhD[a,b,*]

[a]Middleburg Agricultural Research and Extension (MARE) Center,
College of Agriculture and Life Sciences, Virginia Tech,
5527 Sullivans Mill Road, Middleburg, VA 20117, USA
[b]Large Animal Clinical Sciences (0442), Virginia-Maryland Regional College of Veterinary
Medicine, Virginia Polytechnic Institute and State University, Phase II,
Duckpond Drive, 1200 Falcon Ridge Road, Blacksburg, VA 24060, USA

Acute renal failure (ARF) is characterized by an abrupt decrease in glomerular filtration rate (GFR), clinically manifest as a rapid and sustained increase in blood urea and creatinine concentrations together with disturbances to fluid, electrolyte, and acid–base homeostasis [1,2]. The causes of ARF have been classified into three major categories [2]: decreased renal perfusion (prerenal failure), direct renal parenchymal dysfunction (intrinsic renal failure), and obstruction of urine flow or disruption of the lower tract, which leads to accumulation of urine in the abdomen (postrenal failure) (Box 1). In horses, ARF is usually prerenal or renal in origin and is most commonly attributable to hemodynamic or nephrotoxic insults [3]. In neonatal foals, ARF occurs most often as a complication of sepsis, perinatal asphyxial syndrome, or aminoglycoside therapy. With the exception of bladder rupture in the neonate, postrenal failure is rare in the horse.

No data are available on the epidemiology of ARF in horses. Anecdotally, it has been estimated that 0.5% to 1.0% of hospitalized horses have evidence of renal dysfunction. Horses at greatest risk for ARF include those that have acute illness that results in hypovolemia or endotoxemia (eg, colic, colitis, sepsis, exhaustive exercise in warm conditions) or pigmenturia (ie, hemoglobinuria or myoglobinuria), and those that have a history of treatment with potentially nephrotoxic drugs (particularly the aminoglycoside antibiotics and nonsteroidal anti-inflammatory drugs [NSAIDs]) [3]. Evaluation of renal function is warranted in horses that have these conditions because clinical experience has indicated that renal dysfunction is frequently reversible in the early stages of failure. This point has been well illustrated in studies of

---

* Middleburg Agricultural Research and Extension (MARE) Center, 5527 Sullivans Mill Road, Middleburg, VA 20117.

E-mail address: rgeor@vt.edu

0749-0739/07/$ - see front matter © 2007 Elsevier Inc. All rights reserved.
doi:10.1016/j.cveq.2007.09.007
vetequine.theclinics.com

Box 1. Causes of acute renal failure in horses

Prerenal failure
Functional decrease in glomerular filtration rate associated with
   renal hypoperfusion:
   Hypotension or hypovolemia
   Gastrointestinal fluid losses (colic, enterocolitis)
   Acute blood loss
   Exercise-associated sweat losses
   Sepsis/endotoxemia
   Volume redistribution (severe hypoalbuminemia; pleural
      or peritoneal effusion)
   Disseminated intravascular coagulation

Intrinsic Renal Failure
Acute tubular necrosis secondary to:
   Profound or persistent renal hypoperfusion leading to
      ischemic necrosis (continuum from prerenal failure),
      especially in horses receiving nephrotoxic agents in the face
      of inadequate fluid replacement
   Nephrotoxins
      Antimicrobial agents (aminoglycosides, tetracyclines)
      Heavy metals (mercury, arsenic, gold, lead)
      Endogenous substances (myoglobin, hemoglobin)
      Miscellaneous (nonsteroidal anti-inflammatory drugs,
         vitamin D, vitamin K_3 [menadione sodium bisulfite],
         cantharidin, acorns)
Interstitial nephritis or glomerulonephritis secondary to bacterial
   infections (*Leptospirosis pomona*, *Actinobacillus equuli* in
   neonates, sequelae to *Streptococcus equi* infection)

Postrenal failure
Obstructive urolithiasis
Urinary bladder rupture (uroperitoneum) in neonates (rarely in
   postpartum mares)

---

laboratory animals wherein progression from an azotemic state associated
with renal vasoconstriction and intact tubular function (ie, prerenal failure)
to established ARF with tubular dysfunction can be prevented by fluid resuscitation that corrects renal hypoperfusion [4,5].

   This article focuses on the causes and clinical management of ARF in
horses. The pathophysiology of ARF is also briefly discussed, although it
should be recognized that there has been minimal study of ARF in horses
and most information regarding pathophysiologic mechanisms has been
derived from experimental studies in other animal species.

Causes and pathophysiology of acute renal failure

Prerenal or functional renal failure is an appropriate physiologic response to reduced "effective" circulating volume and decreased renal perfusion [6]. Severe or prolonged renal hypoperfusion can result in ischemic injury to the renal tubules and interstitium, however, with resultant development of intrinsic renal failure [7]. Prerenal and intrinsic ARF can therefore be viewed as a continuum of evolving renal dysfunction and injury rather than as separate entities. In horses, hypovolemia associated with gastrointestinal crises (eg, proximal enteritis, colitis, strangulating intestinal obstructions), heavy exercise-associated sweat fluid losses, or profound, acute blood loss could result in decreased renal blood flow and GFR with consequent accumulation of nitrogenous waste products. Sepsis and endotoxemia may also result in reduced effective circulating volume, renal hypoperfusion and prerenal azotemia [8].

True hypovolemia or decreased effective circulating volume invokes systemic and renal responses that, up to a point, preserve renal blood flow and GFR. The decrease in blood pressure activates cardiovascular baroreceptors and initiates activation of the sympathetic nervous system and the renin-angiotensin-aldosterone system, and release of vasopressors, including vasopressin (antidiuretic hormone) and endothelin [6,9]. In the kidney, autoregulatory mechanisms maintain renal blood flow and GFR over a broad range ($\sim$70–160 mm Hg) of mean arterial pressures. Renal autoregulation involves two mechanisms [6,7]. First, there is gradual dilatation of preglomerular (afferent) arterioles mediated by an intrinsic myogenic mechanism (and the influence of prostaglandin I_2 and nitric oxide), with a concomitant constriction of postglomerular (efferent) arterioles under the influence of angiotensin II and other vasopressors. At lower arterial pressures (but still within the range of autoregulation), these responses maintain a fairly constant glomerular capillary hydrostatic pressure. Second, tubuloglomerular feedback serves to regulate and stabilize GFR by feedback from the distal nephron. Increased distal tubular fluid flow results in constriction of afferent arterioles and a decrease in GFR, whereas decreased distal tubular flow results in the opposite effect. This feedback mechanism, which assists with maintaining GFR in the normal range, is mediated by a complex communication between the macula densa and the glomerular microvasculature (see Blantz [6] for review).

Intrinsic ARF may be caused by disorders affecting glomeruli, tubules, interstitium, or vasculature. In human patients, the most common cause of intrinsic ARF is acute tubular dysfunction that results from continuation of the same processes that led to prerenal hypoperfusion. Similarly, in horses tubular dysfunction secondary to prolonged renal hypoperfusion (ischemic injury) is believed to be the most common cause of intrinsic ARF, whereas primary glomerular or interstitial disease is only occasionally recognized. Nephrotoxicity, particularly drug-induced, is also an important cause of intrinsic ARF in horses.

In the human literature, the term acute tubular necrosis (ATN) is frequently used to describe the syndrome of ARF in the absence of prerenal or postrenal azotemia, although this may be a misnomer because necrosis per se may not be a prominent feature of the tubular dysfunction that accompanies intrinsic ARF [4]. A detailed discussion of the pathophysiology is beyond the scope of this article; the reader is referred to recent reviews on this topic [2,4,7,8]. In brief, two factors seem to contribute to the abrupt and sustained decrease in GFR with renal ischemia: (1) a vascular component, including intrarenal vasoconstriction with a decrease in glomerular filtration pressure and vascular congestion of the outer medulla that leads to endothelial cell injury and inflammation; and (2) a tubular component, specifically morphologic changes in the proximal tubules, including loss of polarity, shedding of the brush border, and redistribution of integrins and sodium-potassium ATPase to the apical surface. Increased cytosolic calcium concentration and reactive oxygen species contribute to these morphologic changes and to subsequent cell death and apoptosis. Both viable and nonviable cells are shed into the tubular lumen, resulting in the formation of casts and contributing to the reduction in GFR [4].

The reader is referred elsewhere in this issue for a detailed discussion on toxins affecting the kidneys (see the article by Schmitz elsewhere in this issue). Use of aminoglycoside antibiotics (especially gentamicin) seems to be a common cause of ATN in horses [10–12], and there have been several reports of ARF associated with the administration of NSAIDs, particularly phenylbutazone [10,13]. Aminoglycoside-induced toxicity is the result of damage to proximal tubular epithelial cells [14]. As aminoglycosides are eliminated by the kidney, conditions associated with decreased blood flow or renal function can result in drug accumulation and increased potential for nephrotoxicity. Risk for aminoglycoside nephrotoxicity is therefore probably higher in horses that are dehydrated, hypovolemic, endotoxemic, septic, or hypoxemic. Concurrent use of other potentially nephrotoxic drugs, such as NSAIDs, likely increases the risk for aminoglycoside nephrotoxicity. Similarly, because NSAIDs (either type I or type II cyclooxygenase inhibitors) interfere with autoregulation of renal blood flow and GFR [15,16], risk for nephrotoxicity is increased in patients that have volume depletion or low cardiac output. This increased risk emphasizes the importance of a thorough evaluation of renal function, including measurement of serum urea nitrogen and creatinine concentrations, before initiation of treatment with potentially nephrotoxic agents.

Exposure to endogenous pigments (myoglobin or hemoglobin), heavy metals (mercury-containing counterirritants), or vitamin D or K_3 may also result in intrinsic ARF (see Box 1) [10]. Acute glomerulonephritis (post *Streptococcus equi* infection), interstitial nephritis associated with sepsis (*Actinobacillus equuli* in neonates or *Leptospira* spp infection), or renal microvascular thrombosis (hemolytic uremic-like syndrome) are other less common causes of intrinsic renal failure [3,13]. Myoglobinuric nephrosis can develop secondary to exertional rhabdomyolysis [17], heat stroke, or extensive crush injuries. Causes of intravascular hemolysis and hemoglobinuria include incompatible blood transfusion, immune-mediated hemolytic anemia, fulminant hepatic failure, and toxicosis from ingestion of onions (*Allium* spp) or withered red maple leaves (*Acer rubrum*). In a retrospective study of red maple leaf toxicosis, renal insufficiency was identified in 12 of 30 (41%) horses [18]. Although mechanisms of pigment nephropathy are poorly understood, myoglobin and hemoglobin may decrease renal blood flow and local oxygen tension, with resultant ischemic injury. Tubular obstruction by casts of heme proteins may also contribute to tubular injury. Concurrent hypovolemia and metabolic acidosis may potentiate the development of tubular injury by enhancing free radical formation and lipid peroxidation of cell membranes [2].

Diagnostic evaluation

The diagnostic approach to ARF should include careful evaluation of history (eg, recent administration of potentially nephrotoxic drugs or exposure to other nephrotoxins), a thorough physical examination, and interpretation of laboratory data, including serum biochemistry and examination of urine. In some cases, ultrasonographic examination of the kidneys and renal biopsy may be justified. In horses that have critical illnesses (eg, colitis, systemic inflammatory response syndrome [SIRS]), early diagnosis of renal dysfunction may provide the opportunity to prevent progression from prerenal to established intrinsic ARF.

Clinical examination

In most horses that have ARF, clinical signs are usually referable to the primary problem, such as acute colic, enterocolitis, sepsis, SIRS, or rhabdomyolysis, rather than to renal dysfunction [3,13,19]. In many cases, ARF is only detected when the clinician specifically evaluates renal function through measurement of serum urea nitrogen and creatinine concentrations or urinalysis. In general, the clinical manifestations of ARF reflect the systemic effects of toxic substances usually excreted in the urine (ie, uremia); urinary tract dysfunction (eg, oliguria); and derangements of fluid, electrolyte, and acid–base balance (eg, dehydration). The predominant clinical signs of uremia in horses are depression and anorexia. Rarely, signs of encephalopathy (eg, ataxia, mental obtundation) may also be observed in horses that have severe azotemia [20].

Urine production in horses that have ARF is variable. Oliguria frequently occurs in the early stages of hemodynamically-mediated ARF, but nonoliguric ARF or polyuric ARF may also occur. Polyuria is common during the recovery phase of ARF. Other clinical signs can include dehydration, tachycardia, injected or hyperemic mucous membranes, pyrexia, and mild colic. Colic signs may be more severe in horses that have nephrolithiasis/ureterolithiasis; in these horses, there also may be evidence of hematuria and cystolithiasis. Laminitis, which may be severe and rapidly progressive, is another potential sequela. Transrectal palpation may reveal enlargement of the left kidney and possibly pain on firm palpation; however, this assessment is subjective and normal kidney size does not rule out ARF. Horses that have oliguric renal failure can have perirenal edema that may be detected by palpation per rectum or ultrasonographic examination. Soft feces, attributable to fluid retention, may also be observed in patients that have oliguric ARF. Over a period of 1 to 2 days peripheral edema may also develop because of expansion of interstitial fluid volume, although severe conjunctival edema with prolapse of the ventral conjunctiva and epiphora may be an earlier finding in an occasional horse that has severe acute renal failure.

Laboratory evaluation

Increases in serum or plasma creatinine or urea nitrogen concentrations (ie, azotemia) reflect decreased GFR and should alert the clinician to further investigate the underlying cause and extent of renal dysfunction. It is important to differentiate whether azotemia is predominantly attributable to prerenal failure or intrinsic renal damage. With prerenal failure, volume repletion typically restores renal function and the magnitude of azotemia may decrease by 50% or more during the initial day of treatment. In contrast, with established intrinsic ARF, fluid therapy usually does not lead to prompt resolution of azotemia and, in some cases, serum creatinine concentration continues to increase for a day or two despite intensive fluid therapy and an increase in urine output.

Assessment of urine specific gravity before initiation of fluid therapy is helpful in differentiating prerenal from renal failure. Because normally functioning kidneys would be expected to maximally conserve salt and water in response to a transient decrease in renal blood flow, urine specific gravity is typically greater than 1.035 (and may reach 1.050–1.060) with prerenal failure, whereas urine produced by horses that have intrinsic ARF is often dilute (specific gravity <1.020) because of compromised concentrating ability. Additional measures that can be used to differentiate prerenal failure from intrinsic ARF include fractional sodium clearance and the ratios of urine to serum creatinine concentration and urine to serum osmolality. Intrinsic ARF can be inferred if: (1) the fractional sodium clearance is greater than 1.0%, (2) the ratio of urine to serum creatinine concentration is less than 37 (normal >50), or (3) the ratio of urine osmolality to serum osmolality is less than 1.7 (normal >2.5). One problem with these laboratory assessments is that they are affected by fluid therapy. Application is thus limited to use on urine samples collected before initiation of fluid therapy or the first urine sample voided after fluid therapy has been started. In the clinical situation, assessment of the response to fluid therapy is the most practical way to differentiate prerenal failure from intrinsic renal failure. Azotemia caused by prerenal failure should resolve quickly with replacement of fluid deficits and restoration of renal perfusion. As mentioned, although prerenal failure and intrinsic ARF are often described as two separate entities, the distinction between the two is probably less clear and it is likely that some renal damage occurs in horses that have prerenal failure. Because of the considerable renal reserve capacity, however, renal damage associated with most conditions resulting in transient renal hypoperfusion rarely affects case progression or outcome.

The magnitude of azotemia tends to be lower in nonoliguric ARF than oliguric ARF, possibly indicating less severe injury in nonoliguric ARF. Clinical experience has indicated that nonoliguric ARF is associated with a more favorable prognosis compared with oliguric ARF. In the clinical situation, affected patients are initially treated with large volumes of intravenous fluids for the primary disease (enterocolitis or colic) and oliguria progresses to polyuria. When significant renal damage has been sustained, persistence of oliguric ARF is usually recognized as failure to produce a significant volume of urine in response to fluid therapy, along with minimal change in the degree of azotemia over the initial day of treatment. If these patients are not carefully monitored, fluid retention may lead to development of subcutaneous and pulmonary edema.

The most common electrolyte abnormalities in horses that have ARF, particularly those that have polyuric renal failure, are mild hyponatremia and hypochloremia. Serum potassium concentrations are variable: horses that have oliguric or anuric ARF may have hyperkalemia, whereas those that have polyuric ARF, particularly anorectic patients, may have normokalemia or hypokalemia. With postrenal failure, especially when complicated by uroperitoneum, hyponatremia and hypochloremia are usually more severe and hyperkalemia is commonly found. Hypocalcemia and hyperphosphatemia may be additional findings with ARF [21]. Affected horses often have a degree of metabolic acidosis, especially when ARF is associated with primary problems, such as enterocolitis or severe colic.

As described above, measures of urinary concentrating ability (specific gravity or osmolality) are helpful in assessing development of intrinsic renal failure. Other abnormal urinalysis results can be sensitive indicators of renal damage. This phenomenon is especially true for changes in urine sediment, such as increased numbers of erythrocytes, leukocytes, or presence of casts. Microscopic hematuria, proteinuria, and glucosuria may be additional findings with glomerular or tubular damage. Enzymuria, specifically the ratio of urinary gamma glutamyl transferase (GGT) activity to urinary creatinine (uCr) concentration, has been proposed as a sensitive indicator of renal tubular damage [2]. Because GGT is too large to be filtered by the normal glomerulus and is present in large amounts in the brush border of proximal tubular epithelial cells, a urinary $GGT/(uCr \times 0.01)$ value greater than 25 has been considered to indicate renal tubular disease. Measurement of urinary GGT activity has been advocated for early detection of aminoglyco-side-induced renal disease [22]. This ratio may be falsely elevated in sick horses through a decrease in creatinine excretion, however, consequent to a reduction of GFR. Furthermore, although urinary GGT activity may increase with aminoglycoside therapy, this finding does not necessarily fore-shadow impending renal failure and consequently does not provide useful information regarding the need to either modify the dosing regimen for or discontinue use of aminoglycosides [22].

Although uncommon, acute pyelonephritis can be a cause of ARF and requires submission of a urine sample for quantitative bacterial culture for diagnosis. A history of fever of undetermined origin in a patient that has ARF in the absence of other underlying disease processes should increase suspicion of acute pyelonephritis. In addition, submission of a se-rum sample for determination of titers to *Leptospira* spp serovars may be useful in this type of patient.

Ultrasonography and renal biopsy

Renal ultrasonography using a 3- or 5-MHz sector probe can provide use-ful information regarding renal size and structure. With ARF kidney size may be enlarged and echogenicity of the renal cortices tends to increase resulting in greater distinction between the cortex and medulla (a more prominent cortico-medullary junction) (Fig. 1). Other abnormalities, such as perirenal edema or cystic cavities, may be demonstrated by ultrasonographic examination. Renal ultrasonography may also uncover evidence of underlying chronic renal disease, such as renal hypoplasia or presence of nephroliths, and these findings

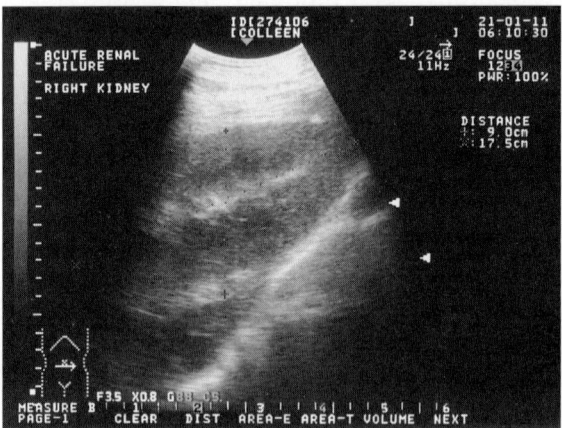

Fig. 1. Ultrasonographic image of the right kidney of a horse that has acute renal failure con-sequent to ingestion of red maple leaves leading to renal ischemia and hemoglobinuria; the kid-ney is enlarged (17.5-cm long axis) and the echogenicity of the renal cortex is increased making the corticomedullary junction more prominent. (*Courtesy of* H. Schott II, DVM, PhD, East Lansing, MI.)

would likely affect prognosis. Percutaneous biopsy of the kidneys is possible in the standing horse, but the technique is not without complications (including perirenal hematoma formation, hematuria, or hemoperitoneum) and is only indicated when a renal mass or other abnormality of renal structure is recognized on ultrasonographic examination. Renal biopsy should also be considered when there is no apparent primary cause for acute renal failure. Ultrasonographic guidance and use of a spring-loaded biopsy instrument (Temno Soft Tissue Biopsy Needle, ProAct Limited, State College, PA) may lessen the risk for complications.

Treatment

Fluid therapy to correct fluid deficits and electrolyte/acid–base abnormalities and promote renal perfusion and urine output is the cornerstone of therapy for ARF, regardless of the cause. Other suggested therapies include diuretics, vasoactive agents, and antioxidants. Renal replacement therapy in the form of hemodialysis [23] or peritoneal dialysis is rarely practical [24].

In horses that have prerenal failure that are at high risk for development of intrinsic ARF, the goal is to prevent or attenuate the pathophysiologic events leading to development of intrinsic renal damage. The primary disease process resulting in prerenal failure must also be identified and appropriately treated. Ideally, administration of nephrotoxic drugs should be discontinued or they should be used sparingly and only when absolutely indicated for treatment of the primary disease. For situations in which continued administration of aminoglycoside antibiotics or NSAIDs is necessary, alterations in dosing regimens may lessen the risk for renal injury. With regard to the aminoglycosides, monitoring serum drug concentrations allows the clinician to individualize dosage regimens. For example, the risk for nephrotoxicity with aminoglycosides increases when trough concentrations remain high (>2 μg/mL for gentamicin or >5 μg/mL for amikacin) [25]. Serum trough concentrations can be reduced below these values by increasing the dosage interval. When therapy with NSAIDs is continued, the minimally effective dose should be used. Combinations of potentially nephrotoxic drugs (eg, an aminoglycoside and an NSAID) should be limited and there is no indication for simultaneous use of multiple NSAIDs.

Blood samples for biochemical and acid–base analyses should be submitted before initiation of therapy. In addition, packed cell volume, plasma total solids, and body weight should be determined. Although frequently overlooked, daily recording of body weight is perhaps the best measure of fluid balance in horses that have fluid loss/retention and renal dysfunction. Measurement of body weight is also critical for correct determination of drug dosages. Estimated fluid deficit should be replaced over the first 12 hours of treatment. If serum potassium concentration is elevated (>4.5 mEq/L), physiologic saline (0.9% NaCl solution) is the fluid of choice unless hypernatremia is present, in which case a 0.45% NaCl/2.5% dextrose solution can be used. If serum potassium concentration is normal, a polyionic replacement fluid (eg, lactated Ringer's solution, Plasmalyte, or Normosol-R) could also be used because the amount of potassium that would be administered over the initial 12 hours would likely be less than 1% of total body potassium content. The estimated fluid deficit can be calculated by multiplying the estimated dehydration (%) by body weight (kg). For example, for a 500-kg horse that is 8% dehydrated: 0.08×500 kg $= 40$ kg $= 40$ liters.

In horses that have prerenal failure, renal perfusion, GFR, and urine output (15–30 mL/kg/day) should return to normal after correction of the fluid deficit. Although most horses that have some degree of intrinsic ARF increase urine production in response to fluid therapy, a few patients may remain oliguric after correction of fluid deficits and these horses must be closely monitored for signs of overhydration. Ideally, central venous pressure (normal values are <8 cm H_2O) would be monitored in patients that have oliguric ARF. Daily measurement of body weight, packed cell volume, and plasma total solids; observation of respiratory rate and effort and auscultation of the lungs for sounds consistent with pulmonary edema; and observation for the development of dependent edema are more practical means to assess hydration state. Pulmonary edema can develop rapidly in horses that have severe oliguric ARF; clinical experience has shown that as little as 40 mL/kg of intravenous (IV) fluids (20 L for a 500-kg horse) may result in pulmonary edema in these patients.

With the exception of horses that have severe oliguric ARF or postrenal failure, serum potassium concentration is usually within normal limits and specific therapy intended to lower serum potassium concentration is not required. In select cases, however, recognition and treatment of hyperkalemia is essential because increases in serum potassium concentrations (to 6.5–8.0 mEq/L) have the potential to induce cardiac arrhythmias (bradycardia, atrial standstill, ventricular tachycardia). Moderate hyperkalemia usually resolves in response to administration of potassium-free fluids and improved urine flow. Horses that have severe hyperkalemia (>7.0 mEq/L) and cardiac arrhythmias should be treated with agents that decrease serum potassium concentration (sodium bicarbonate, 1–2 mEq/kg IV over 5 to 15 minutes) or counteract the effects of hyperkalemia on cardiac conduction (calcium gluconate, 0.5 mL/kg of a 10% solution by slow IV injection or added to 5 L of IV fluids and administered over 1 hour).

Drug treatments to increase renal perfusion or urine production

Furosemide (1.0–2.0 mg/kg IV, every 6 hours, or as a constant rate infusion), dopamine (3–5 µg/kg/min IV, in a 5% dextrose solution), and mannitol (0.25–1.0 g/kg as a 20% solution administered IV over 15 to 20 minutes) have all been advocated for treatment of oliguric ARF refractory to volume replacement therapy [26]. The goal of these treatments is to increase renal perfusion and urine production by renal vasodilation, diuresis, or a combination of these mechanisms. It must be emphasized, however, that the efficacy of these treatments has not been assessed in horses that have ARF and, particularly for mannitol and dopamine, the risk for adverse effects associated with the administration of these agents likely outweighs any theoretic benefit. In human medicine, recent critical reviews on the management of ARF have concluded that there are no data to support the use of dopamine or mannitol [27–29], whereas the effect of loop diuretics on clinical outcome have been equivocal [30,31].

Furosemide and other loop diuretics may reduce oxygen demand in the medullary thick ascending loop of Henle by blocking the Na+/K+/2Cl– cotransporter in the luminal membrane, with a concomitant decrease in Na+/K+-ATPase activity in the basolateral membrane [27]. Timely administration of loop diuretics might therefore attenuate ischemic damage of tubular cells and reduce the severity of ARF. Loop diuretics may have a further benefit in patients that have ARF by increasing urine output [27]. In equine practice, furosemide is commonly used in an attempt to convert oliguric to nonoliguric ARF. Urine output of horses that have oliguric ARF following administration of the drug seems to vary widely but most clinicians report that the drug has rarely been effective in converting oliguric ARF to nonoliguric ARF. The effect of furosemide on urine flow depends on intact proximal tubular secretion and tubular flow for delivery of the drug to the active site in the lumen of the medullary thick ascending limb [27]. Acute tubular necrosis and tubular obstruction with cellular debris and pigments can thus limit delivery of furosemide to the active site. Taken together, these mechanisms may contribute to the variable and often poor diuretic response in horses that have oliguric ARF. It is noteworthy that in human patients who have ARF, furosemide treatment does not affect long-term outcome and in two meta-analysis studies was not associated with any significant clinical benefit [30,31]. Nevertheless, furosemide continues to be used in many horses that have oliguric ARF on the basis of occasional anecdotal reports of apparent conversion of oliguric to nonoliguric renal failure. Because furosemide administration has been demonstrated to exacerbate gentamicin toxicity in other species [27], its use is probably ill advised in horses that have ARF secondary to aminoglycoside usage.

When furosemide is used in horses that have oliguria, an initial dose of 1 to 2 mg/kg IV should be administered. If an increase in urine output is not observed after 45 to 60 minutes, a larger dose (4–6 mg/kg IV) can be administered. Higher doses of furosemide may overcome the limitations in tubular drug delivery associated with the administration of more standard intravenous doses. If an increase in urine production is observed, furosemide administration should be continued at 1 to 3 mg/kg IV two to three times daily until clinical improvement is observed (eg, partial resolution of azotemia). As an alternative, furosemide can also be administered as a continuous rate infusion to have continuous, rather than episodic, delivery of furosemide to the kidneys. Obviously, IV fluid therapy must be continued during the period of furosemide treatment to avoid exacerbation of hypovolemia. Electrolyte and acid–base status should also be monitored at regular intervals during therapy.

Anecdotally, dopamine has been widely used in the management of horses that have ARF. There have also been reports of the administration of dopamine infusions to dehydrated, hypovolemic endurance horses, even before institution of adequate IV fluid replacement. It has been suggested that this treatment may attenuate renal injury associated with hypoperfusion. Studies in healthy horses have demonstrated a dose-dependent increase in renal blood flow with administration of dopamine [32]. At low doses (1–3 µg/kg/min), this response likely reflects the renal arteriolar vasodilation by stimulation of dopamine receptors (subtype DA-1) on intrarenal vessels. At moderate doses (3–5 µg/kg/min), an increase in renal perfusion may be attributable to inotropy (by stimulation of β-receptors), whereas at high doses (5–20 µg/kg/min) the enhanced renal blood flow may be attributable to increased perfusion pressure (by stimulation of α_1-adrenoceptors) [33]. Studies in human subjects have indicated that the effects of dopamine on systemic and renal hemodynamics are unpredictable and, even at the low dose, dopamine infusion may result in systemic vasoconstriction and decreased renal perfusion [27]. Large randomized controlled trials have shown low-dose dopamine to lack efficacy on renal outcome or overall mortality in human patients who have ARF [34]. Recent literature on the clinical management of ARF in critically ill human patients has advocated abandonment of routine use of low-dose dopamine [34,35]. Similarly, there is insufficient evidence to support the use of dopamine in the management of ARF in horses.

Administration of mannitol (1 g/kg IV over 30–60 min), an osmotic agent, increases plasma osmolality and induces fluid shifts that increase effective circulating volume, renal blood flow, and GFR [27]. In the kidney, the osmotic effects of mannitol also may enhance tubular flow and urine output. The osmotic diuresis induced by mannitol may also increase renal tubular oxygen demand, however, thereby increasing susceptibility to ischemic injury. In other species there is evidence that high doses of mannitol (3 g/kg) exacerbate ARF [27]. For these reasons, mannitol is no longer recommended in the management of oliguric ARF in human patients. It should be further noted that use of an osmotic diuretic agent is contraindicated in overhydrated patients because the associated increase in intravascular volume may precipitate or exacerbate pulmonary edema.

Adjunct therapies and clinical monitoring

Once volume deficits have been corrected and diuresis has been established, fluid therapy should be tailored to provide for maintenance requirements. The author uses 55 to 60 mL/kg/d (or 1 L/h to a 400–500 kg horse) as an estimate of daily fluid requirements for adult horses. During the polyuric recovery phase of ARF, however, urine volume and urinary electrolyte losses can be greater than normal, and maintenance fluid requirements may need to be increased. Potassium supplementation (20–40 mEq of KCl added to each liter of IV fluids) may also be necessary, particularly for anorectic patients. An estimate of the volume of ongoing fluid losses for the primary disease process (enterocolitis) should also be included in the daily plan for fluid administration. Polyionic fluids, such as lactated Ringer's solution, should be used once electrolyte and acid–base alterations have been corrected. Oral electrolyte therapy (eg, 30 g NaCl once or twice daily, administered as slurry by way of dosing syringe) is also useful for encouragement of water consumption and urine output. In normokalemic, anorectic horses, the administration of potassium chloride (15–30 g by mouth twice daily) is also indicated.

Protracted ARF and anorexia can lead to a catabolic state and affected patients often require nutritional support. Adding dextrose to IV fluids (5%–10% solution) may provide some nutritional support, but the calories provided do not meet minimum daily requirements and parenteral nutrition solutions containing protein and lipids may be indicated. Critical illness and protracted inanition can also increase the risk for gastric ulceration. Treatment with omeprazole (2–4 mg/kg by mouth every 24 hours) or cimetidine (8–10 mg/kg IV every 8 hours) may therefore be warranted.

Frequent patient monitoring is essential to assess response to therapy. The minimum data collected on a daily basis should include clinical assessment, body weight, packed cell volume, plasma total solids, serum concentrations of creatinine and electrolytes, and volume of fluid administered. Intravenous fluid therapy should be continued until the horse is eating and drinking normally and there has been a substantial decrease (>75%) in creatinine concentration. The volume of fluids administered should be reduced gradually over a 2- to 3-day period before discontinuing fluid therapy. It is important to monitor the patient's hydration status during this period. The serum creatinine concentration should be measured again 2 to 3 days after fluid therapy is discontinued.

Prognosis

The prognosis for ARF in the horse depends on the underlying cause, duration of renal failure, response to initial treatment, and development of secondary complications, such as laminitis, thrombophlebitis, and diarrhea. Regardless of the cause, the duration of renal failure before initiation of treatment is the most important determinant of prognosis. Early interruption of the pathophysiologic events that lead to ARF provides the best chance of preventing permanent renal dysfunction. Horses that have hemodynamically mediated ARF secondary to conditions such as diarrhea, endotoxemia, hemolytic crises, and myopathy usually have a fair to good prognosis for full recovery of renal function provided that appropriate therapy is instituted and the primary problem can be corrected.

The expected response to therapy in patients that have prerenal failure (serum creatinine concentration typically <5 mg/dL) is rapid resolution of azotemia over the first 2 to 3 days of treatment. Patients that have a favorable prognosis for recovery from intrinsic ARF (serum creatinine concentration may range from 5–10 mg/dL) have a more gradual decline in serum creatinine concentration over a 3- to 7-day period, although complete resolution of azotemia may take 4 to 6 weeks. A more guarded prognosis should be given for patients that have a serum creatinine concentration greater than 10 mg/dL at initial evaluation and when azotemia is unchanged or worse after the first day or two of treatment. The prognosis is poor for horses that have more severe azotemia at initial evaluation (creatinine concentration >15 mg/dL) and for those that remain oliguric 24 to 48 hours after the start of intensive treatment. In these horses, a high incidence of secondary complications, such as generalized edema and laminitis, contributes to the poor prognosis.

Summary

Acute renal failure in horses is usually prerenal or renal in origin and most often caused by hemodynamic or nephrotoxic insults. The clinical management of patients that have ARF is largely supportive, including correction of fluid deficits and electrolyte and acid–base disturbances and treatment and reversal of the underlying cause. Use of dopamine and mannitol to promote renal blood flow and urine output is no longer recommended.

References

[1] Hilton R. Acute renal failure. Br Med J 2006;333:786–90.
[2] Lameire N, Van Biesen W, Vanholder R. Acute renal failure. Lancet 2005;365:417–30.
[3] Geor RJ. Acute renal failure. In: Robinson NE, editor. Current therapy in equine medicine 5. Philadelphia: Saunders; 2003. p. 839–44.
[4] Schrier RW, Wang W, Poole B, et al. Acute renal failure: definitions, diagnosis, pathogenesis and therapy. J Clin Invest 2004;114:5–14.
[5] Reineck HJ, O'Connor GJ, Lifschitz MD, et al. Sequential studies on the pathophysiology of glycerol-induced acute renal failure. J Lab Clin Med 1980;96:356–262.
[6] Blantz RC. Pathophysiology of pre-renal azotemia. Kidney Int 1998;53:512–23.
[7] Kribben A, Edelstein CL, Schrier RW. Pathophysiology of acute renal failure. J Nephrol 1999;12(Suppl 2):S142–51.
[8] Schrier RW, Wang W. Acute renal failure and sepsis. N Engl J Med 2004;351:159–69.
[9] Badr KF, Ichikawa I. Prerenal failure: a deleterious shift from renal compensation to decompensation. N Engl J Med 1988;319:623–9.
[10] Schmitz DG. Toxic nephropathy in horses. Compend Cont Educ Pract Vet 1988;10:104–11.
[11] Bartol JM, Divers TJ, Perkins GA. Case presentation: Nephrotoxicant-induced acute renal failure in five horses. Compend Cont Educ Pract Vet 2000;22:870–6.
[12] Riviere JE, Traver DS, Coppoc GL. Gentamicin toxic nephropathy in horses with disseminated bacterial infection. J Am Vet Med Assoc 1982;180:648–51.

[13] Bayly WM. Acute renal failure. In: Reed SM, Bayly WM, Sellon DC, editors. Equine internal medicine. 2nd edition. St. Louis (MO): Saunders; 2004. p. 1221–30.

[14] Riviere JE, Coppoc GL. Selected aspects of aminoglycoside antibiotic nephrotoxicosis. J Am Vet Med Assoc 1981;178:508–9.

[15] Brater DC. Anti-inflammatory agents and renal function. Semin Arthritis Rhem 2002; 32(Suppl 1):33–42.

[16] Gambaro G, Perazella MA. Adverse renal effects of anti-inflammatory agents: evaluation of selective and nonselective cyclooxygenase inhibitors. J Intern Med 2003;253:643–52.

[17] Sprayberry KA, Madigan J, LeCouteur RA, et al. Renal failure, laminitis, and colitis following severe rhabdomyolysis in a draft-cross with polysaccharide storage myopathy. Can Vet J 1998;39:500–3.

[18] Alward A, Corriher CA, Barton MH, et al. Red maple (Acer rubrum) leaf toxicity in horses: a retrospective study of 32 cases. J Vet Intern Med 2006;20:1197–201.

[19] Divers TJ, Whitlock RH, Byars TD, et al. Acute renal failure in six horses resulting from hemodynamic causes. Equine Vet J 1987;19:178–84.

[20] Frye MA, Johnson JS, Traub-Dargatz JL, et al. Putative uremic encephalopathy in horses: five cases (1978–1998). J Am Vet Med Assoc 2001;218:560–6.

[21] Elfer RS, Bayly WM, Brobst DF, et al. Alterations in calcium, phosphorus and C-terminal parathyroid levels in equine acute renal disease. Cornell Vet 1986;76:317–29.

[22] Rossier Y, Divers TJ, Sweeney RW. Variations in urinary gamma glutamyl transferase/urinary creatinine ratio in horses with or without pleuropneumonia treated with gentamicin. Equine Vet J 1995;27:217–20.

[23] Vivrette S, Cowgill LD, Pascoe J, et al. Hemodialysis for treatment of oxytetracycline-induced acute renal failure in a neonatal foal. J Am Vet Med Assoc 1993;203:105–7.

[24] Gallatin LL, Couetil LL, Ash SR. Use of continuous-flow peritoneal dialysis for the treatment of acute renal failure in an adult horse. J Am Vet Med Assoc 2005;226:756–9.

[25] Geor RJ, Papich MG. Once-daily aminoglycoside dosing regimens. In: Robinson NE, editor. Current therapy in equine medicine 5. Philadelphia: Saunders; 2003. p. 850–3.

[26] Jose-Cunilleras E, Hinchcliff KW. Renal pharmacology. Vet Clin North Am Equine Pract 1999;15:647–64.

[27] Dishart MK, Kellum JA. An evaluation of pharmacological strategies for the prevention and treatment of acute renal failure. Drugs 2000;59:79–91.

[28] Lameire NH, De Vriese AS, Vanholder R. Prevention and nondialytic treatment of acute renal failure. Curr Opin Crit Care 2003;9:481–90.

[29] Fry AC, Farrington K. Management of acute renal failure. Postgrad Med 2006;82:106–16.

[30] Bagshaw SM, Delaney A, Haase M, et al. Loop diuretics in the management of acute renal failure: a systematic review and meta-analysis. Crit Care Resusc 2007;9:60–8.

[31] Ho KM, Sheridan DJ. Meta-analysis of frusemide to prevent or treat acute renal failure. Brit Med J, doi:10.1136/bmj.38902.605347.7 C (published 21 July 2006).

[32] Trim CM, Moore JN, Clark ES. Renal effects of dopamine infusion in conscious horses. Equine Vet J 1989;(Suppl 7):124–8.

[33] Denton MD, Chertow GM, Brady HR. "Renal-dose" dopamine for the treatment of acute renal failure: scientific rationale, experimental studies, and clinical trials. Kidney Int 1996;49: 4–14.

[34] Lauschke A, Teichgraber UKM, Frie U, et al. 'Low-dose' dopamine worsens renal perfusion in patients with acute renal failure. Kidney Int 2006;69:1669–74.

[35] Jones D, Bellomo R. Renal-dose dopamine: from hypothesis to paradigm to dogma to myth, and, finally superstition. J Intensive Care Med 2005;20:199–211.

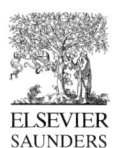

VETERINARY
CLINICS
Equine Practice

Vet Clin Equine 23 (2007) 593–612

ELSEVIER
SAUNDERS

Chronic Renal Failure in Horses

Harold C. Schott II, DVM, PhD

*Department of Large Animal Clinical Sciences, College of Veterinary Medicine, D-202
Veterinary Medical Center, Michigan State University, East Lansing, MI 48824–1314, USA*

Chronic renal failure (CRF) is a syndrome of progressive loss of renal function that results in loss of urinary concentrating ability, retention of nitrogenous and other metabolic end products, alterations in electrolyte and acid-base status, and dysfunction of several hormone systems [1,2]. Retention of organic waste products normally excreted in urine leads to alterations in cell membrane integrity and cellular function. Further, endocrine functions of the kidney (ie, production of erythropoietin and the active form of vitamin D) are diminished and clearance times for hormones (eg, gastrin and parathormone) eliminated by renal excretion may be prolonged. Ultimately, a clinical syndrome of multiple organ dysfunction, termed "uremia," develops [3]. However, clinical signs of uremia are nonspecific and include lethargy, inappetance, and weight loss. In horses, CRF is only one diagnosis on a long list of causes of "ill thrift" and weight loss [4] and, unfortunately, a diagnosis of CRF is often not established until the condition has progressed to end-stage renal disease (ESRD).

Classically, loss of concentrating ability develops in mammals when two thirds of nephron function has been lost and this syndrome, in the absence of azotemia, has been called either "renal insufficiency" or "compromised renal function." With loss of three fourths or more of nephron function, azotemia, a laboratory term for increased blood concentrations of urea (BUN) and creatinine (Cr), develops [1,2]. Loss of varying degrees of renal function in association with these fractional losses of kidney tissue has been determined in experimental studies in several mammalian species subjected to nephrectomy of one kidney and subtotal nephrectomy of the contralateral kidney [5,6]. Although these models of CRF have provided considerable information for the understanding of CRF, it is important to recognize that experimental models are not always comparable with the loss of renal function with spontaneously occurring renal disease. Specifically, with naturally occurring renal disease damage to nephrons is rarely distributed

E-mail address: schott@cvm.msu.edu

homogeneously throughout the kidneys and less or unaffected nephrons may develop compensatory changes in function by increasing glomerular size and single nephron glomerular filtration rate (GFR). Although increasing single nephron GFR may be useful for increased filtration and excretion of waste products, this compensatory response can also be accompanied by increases in glomerular capillary hydrostatic pressure; activation of the renin-angiotensin-aldosterone system ([RAAS] leading to hypertension); and increased filtration of proteins across the glomerular basement membrane (GBM). Unfortunately, these consequences are ultimately counterproductive and contribute to the progressive deterioration of renal function that is a hallmark of CRF [5–8].

The progressive nature of CRF is manifested by a slow decline in renal function over a period of months to years. Further loss of renal function can be attenuated, however, by interventions made once the initial diagnosis has been established. In human medicine, CRF represents a substantial economic challenge to the health care system because an inordinate amount of resources are currently being used on a proportionately smaller fraction of the patient population with ESRD that requires dialysis or is awaiting renal transplantation [9]. Considerable effort is being directed both at recognizing earlier stages of chronic kidney disease (CKD) and developing management strategies that slow progression and prolong the interval from initial diagnosis of CKD to the need for renal replacement therapy. A substantial aspect of this effort is identification and appropriate management of hypertension and diabetes, conditions that are major risk factors for development of CKD [10]. Similarly, in small animal medicine recent efforts have also focused on early recognition of CKD and management strategies (eg, renal diets and medications) both to improve quality of life and prolong survival for affected dogs and cats [11–13]. Although equine medicine is lagging a bit behind these efforts in other species, when CRF is recognized in its earlier stages in equine patients, perhaps during evaluation for other problems, affected horses can be managed successfully for months to years.

This article describes the prevalence, causes, clinical signs, diagnostic evaluation, and management of horses afflicted with CRF. It is hoped that this article illustrates that CRF, when detected in the earlier stages of disease, can be managed successfully in the short-term allowing owners to enjoy a period of time of ongoing productivity, performance, or companionship until loss of condition reaches the point that euthanasia becomes warranted.

Prevalence of chronic renal failure

Fortunately, CRF is an uncommon problem in horses. The prevalence of CRF was reported to be 0.9% and 1.6% for dogs and cats, respectively, in 1990 [1]. Compared with prior years, the prevalence in dogs remained stable, whereas the occurrence of CRF in cats seems to be on the increase, especially in older patients. Data retrieved from the Veterinary Medical database at

Purdue University yielded 515 of 442,535 horses admitted to participating veterinary teaching hospitals during the years 1964 through 1996 with a diagnosis of CRF (prevalence of 0.12%) [2]. This is probably an underestimate because euthanasia was likely performed in a number of cases of chronic weight loss without a definitive diagnosis being established and without presentation to a veterinary teaching hospital. As in small animals, CRF seems to be a greater problem in older horses: the prevalence increased to 0.23% in horses older than 15 years. A prevalence of 0.51% for intact males over 15 years of age could also suggest that stallions are at greater risk for developing CRF. An alternate explanation for an apparently higher prevalence in older stallions may simply be, however, that their greater value led to increased likelihood of diagnosis and attempt at management of the syndrome. In a group of 467 geriatric horses (20 years or older) presented to a veterinary teaching hospital from 1989 to 1999, 13 (3%) were presented for evaluation of disorders of the urinary tract [14]. In this report, five horses had squamous cell carcinoma of the penis but the number of horses that may have been afflicted with CRF was not detailed. If four to five of these older horses had CRF, the prevalence would have been approximately 1%.

Pathophysiology and causes of chronic renal failure

Limited work in horses suggests that they are similar to other mammals in terms of loss of kidney function with loss of renal functional mass. Normal horses subjected to unilateral nephrectomy experienced transient increases in BUN and Cr but renal function, as assessed by this routine clinicopathologic assessment, returned to normal within several days following nephrectomy (R. DeBowes, personal communication, 1991). Further, these experimental horses maintained body condition and weight for the remainder of the time they were observed following nephrectomy. Long-term survival following unilateral nephrectomy for treatment of a number of renal disorders also supports that horses remain largely unaffected by loss of 50% of renal functional mass [15–20]. In other mammals studied, hypertrophy of the remnant kidney is commonly observed, especially when nephrectomy is performed in young animals [6]. The author has also observed enlargement of the contralateral kidney following diagnosis of unilateral renal disease treated with or without nephrectomy. Collectively, these observations suggest that the equine kidney adapts to nephron loss in a similar manner as in other mammals with compensatory partial restoration of lost renal function.

Natural causes of CRF in horses generally can be grouped into anomalies of development; immune-mediated disorders primarily affecting glomeruli (glomerulonephritis [GN]) and less commonly tubular and interstitial structures; and tubulointerstitial disease termed "chronic interstitial nephritis" (CIN). In a review of 99 horses with CRF, signalment included a number of breeds but the three breeds most commonly affected were Thoroughbreds (29%), Standardbreds (10%), and Clydesdales (10%) [21]. Sex distribution included 44% mares, 40% geldings, and 16% stallions. Of interest, one third of all cases occurred in horses that were less than 6 years of age and congenital renal disorders were found in 16% of horses. Anomalies reported included renal agenesis, renal hypoplasia, renal dysplasia, and polycystic kidney disease (PCKD). Acquired disease was the cause of CRF in the remaining cases (84%). Approximately one half of the acquired cases were attributed to GN (53%) and the remainder had CIN (39%) or ESRD (8%). It should be emphasized that this case series was compiled by combining 29 clinical cases examined by the author with 70 previously reported cases. Based on a substantially higher incidence of CIN than GN in the 29 clinical cases, it is probable that GN has been overrepresented in previous reports. In the author's experience, primary GN seems to be rare and is likely responsible for development of CRF in less than 10% of affected equids.

Anomalies of development

Congenital disorders that may cause CRF include renal agenesis and hypoplasia, renal dysplasia, PCKD, and other glomerular or tubular disorders. Complete renal agenesis is clearly incompatible with life and affected neonates die within the first few days of life [22]. Horses with unilateral renal agenesis or renal hypoplasia are born with less renal functional mass but may never develop any clinical evidence of renal insufficiency as long as they have 30% to 40% of a normal number of functional nephrons. Horses with these anomalies are certainly at greater risk of developing CRF, however, if they are challenged by other disorders (eg, colic or enterocolitis) that can be accompanied by a degree of acute renal failure (ARF) and use of potentially nephrotoxic medications leading to some loss of functional nephrons. Renal dysplasia is a disorder in which both glomeruli and tubules fail to form normally during embryologic development. The consequences are glomeruli of variable size and development and tubules that vary from near normal in structure to blind-ending structures that are nonfunctional. Most cases of renal dysplasia have been reported in horses less than 1 year of age [23–27] but affected individuals have also survived for several years before CRF has been recognized [28,29].

PCKD has been reported in a limited number of equids [30–34]. In people, Bull Terrier dogs, and Persian cats, PCKD is recognized to be a genetic disease with both dominant and recessive modes of inheritance [35–39]. Although a genetic disorder, affected patients often remain healthy until adulthood because renal function remains adequate. Over the first few months to years of life cystic structures within the kidneys slowly enlarge leading to a progressive decline in renal function. In some instances the kidneys increase dramatically in size, whereas with other forms of the disease the kidneys are not grossly enlarged but contain multiple, variable-sized cysts. Ultrasonographic imaging of the kidneys can be used to screen at-risk animals after the initial 9 months of life [40]. Although the anomaly is uncommon in horses and no familial occurrence has yet been described, it is logical to consider a genetic basis for PCKD in horses. As an example, the author recently evaluated a 19-year-old Arabian mare with CRF attributable to PCKD (Fig. 1). Ultrasonographic imaging of the mare's 2-month-old foal revealed normal renal size and architecture but it is possible that PCKD could develop over time in one or more of the mare's offspring.

Although there have been no reports in horses to date, familial glomerulopathies and tubular disorders have been reported in people and dogs (Bull Terrier hereditary nephritis, comparable with Alport's syndrome in people caused by a defect in collagen type IV) [41,42] and cattle (renal tubular dysplasia in Japanese Black cattle) [43]. These anomalies of development can spread rapidly within certain breeds when accompanied by other desired phenotypical characteristics and dominant modes of inheritance (similar to hyperkalemic periodic paralysis in Quarter Horses).

In horses, anomalies of development should be suspected in patients with CRF that are less than 10 years of age and for which no history of risk factors (eg, prior disorders accompanied by prolonged hypovolemia or requiring treatment with nephrotoxic drugs) exists. Unfortunately, long-term histories for many horses are unknown because of changes in ownership and a lack of continuity of medical records.

Glomerulonephritis

Glomerular injury leading to focal glomerular disease seems to be a relatively common lesion in horses; however, progression to clinical CRF

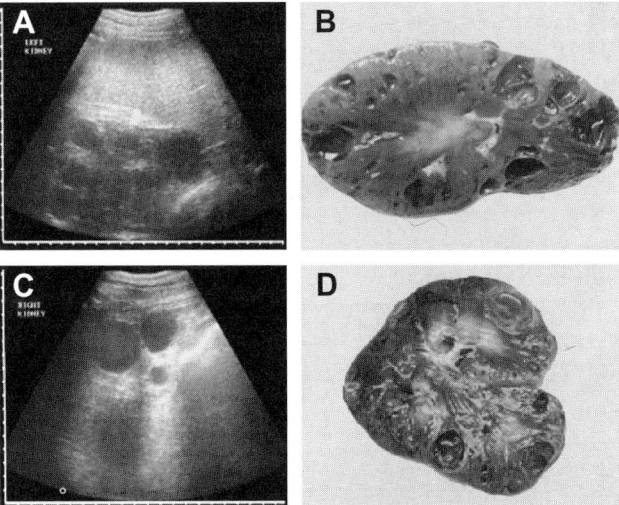

Fig. 1. Ultrasonographic images of the left (A) and right (C) kidneys and cross sectional gross pathology of the left (B) and right (D) kidneys of a 19-year-old Arabian mare with chronic renal failure attributablet to polycystic kidney disease.

remains a rare event. In one postmortem study, 16% of 45 horses examined had glomerular lesions on light microscopy and 42% (22 of 53 horses examined) exhibited deposits containing immunoglobulin or complement on immunofluorescence staining [44]. Although these findings suggest that as many as one third of horses may show microscopic evidence of renal disease, only one of the horses in this survey exhibited signs of CRF. In addition to immune-mediated injury, integrity of the glomerular barrier can also be disrupted by other disease processes, including ischemia, toxic insults, and infection [45]. These mechanisms usually lead to significant vascular and tubulointerstitial changes in addition to glomerular injury.

Use of the term GN is typically reserved to describe renal disease in which immune-mediated glomerular damage is suspected to be the initiating factor in development of renal failure. The hallmark of GN is increased permeability of the glomerular barrier characterized by proteinuria and microscopic (and occasionally macroscopic) hematuria [46]. Light microscopic examination may reveal hypercellularity of the glomerular tufts (proliferative GN) or thickening of the glomerular barrier (membranous GN). Examination of the GBM by electron microscopy reveals thickening of the glomerular barrier and scattered electron dense deposits in the GBM. Immunohistochemical staining with antiequine immunoglobulin antibodies may reveal immunofluorescence in a scattered or "lumpy-bumpy" pattern, consistent with immune complex deposition in the GBM [2,44,46].

In horses, chronic infections leading to a prolonged period in which circulating immune complexes could be deposited in the GBM are most likely to result in GN. For example, experimental *Leptospira pomona* infection produced subacute GN characterized by hypercellularity and edema of capillary tufts [47], but leptospirosis is a rare cause of clinical renal disease in horses [48,49]. Similarly, experimental infection with equine infectious anemia virus produced histologic and immunofluorescent evidence of GN in 75% and 87% of infected horses, respectively, and equine infectious anemia viral antigens were eluted from the GBM [50]. Clinical renal disease was not observed, however, in any of the experimentally infected horses. Poststreptococcal GN is a well-recognized cause of CKD in humans [51] and *Streptococcus equi* subspecies zooepidemicus and subspecies *equi* are common causes of chronic infection in horses. In one report, development of GN in a horse with chronic pleuritis and purpura hemorrhagica was speculated to be a consequence of circulating immune complexes involving streptococcal antigens [52]. Further, immune complexes comprised of group-C streptococcal antigen and IgG were identified in the GBM of a horse with CRF that had a history of prior respiratory disease from which *S equi* subspecies zooepidemicus had been isolated [53]. An occasional case of equine GN may also be a consequence of true autoimmune disease in which autoantibodies are directed against GBM antigens and immunofluorescent staining reveals a more diffuse or linear pattern along the GBM [44]. Similarly, a recent report of a horse with chronic ill thrift and moderate to severe proteinuria revealed immunoreactivity to IgM in the GBM but no evidence for an inciting infectious agent could be found [54]. Finally, although GN seems to be an uncommon inciting cause of CRF in horses, subclinical GN likely goes unrecognized in many patients. For example, the author has observed hematuria and proteinuria in a few horses with purpura hemorrhagica but CRF has not developed in these patients.

Chronic interstitial nephritis

CIN is somewhat of a catch-all term for diseases starting in the tubules or interstitium. Although supportive data are lacking, tubulointerstitial disease is usually considered a consequence of acute tubular necrosis (ATN) secondary to ischemia, sepsis, or exposure to nephrotoxic compounds [55–59]. Aminoglycoside antibiotics, nonsteroidal anti-inflammatory drugs, vitamin D, vitamin K_3, acorns, and heavy metals, such as mercury, are all potentially nephrotoxic. Intravascular hemolysis or rhabdomyolysis can also lead to ATN secondary to the nephrotoxic effects of hemoglobin or myoglobin [59]. CRF may develop as a sequela to prior ATN with or without a history of clinical ARF. Because of changes in ownership and lack of extensive medical histories for many equine patients, knowledge about disorders that may have caused prior renal damage and ARF is often unavailable when horses are presented for evaluation of CRF. Of interest, data describing the impact of prior ARF on subsequent development of CKD in people are also limited. The United States Renal Data System listed "acute tubular necrosis without recovery" as the cause of ESRD in only 1% to 2% of patients between 1994 and 2003 [60]. The mortality of ARF consequent to ATN that develops in human intensive care units remains high (approximately 50%), however, and hypertension and diabetes are considerably greater risk factors for development of CRF in people as compared with horses. Although it is possible that a greater percentage of horses that develop CRF experienced a significant renal insult months to years previously, such a history has been absent for most cases of CRF attributable to CIN seen by the author.

CIN culminating in CRF can also be caused by ascending urinary tract infection resulting in pyelonephritis [61–64] or complicated by obstructive disease caused by ureterolithiasis or nephrolithiasis [65,66]. Upper tract lithiasis is a common finding in horses with CIN [66,67]. These uroliths are composed of calcium carbonate crystals that are deposited and grow at sites of renal parenchymal damage. Unlike nephrolithiasis in people in which stones are often the primary problem [68], upper tract stones should be considered a secondary problem in horses, rather than a cause of renal disease. Nephroliths that accompany CIN are frequently found bilaterally but they are rarely obstructive; consequently, removal is not indicated unless they are considered a cause of recurrent renal colic or a focus of persistent sepsis (or when they are truly obstructive causing hydronephrosis). Finally, although not yet described in horses, immune mechanisms, including anti–tubular basement membrane disease, can lead to CIN in humans [69].

End-stage renal disease

ESRD describes the severe gross and histologic changes in kidneys collected from animals in the final stages of CRF. Grossly, the kidneys are pale, shrunken, and firm, and they may have an irregular surface and an adherent capsule. Histologically, severe glomerulosclerosis and extensive interstitial fibrosis are observed. The end-stage lesions make it virtually impossible to determine the inciting cause of renal disease.

Other causes of chronic renal failure

Several early reports of CRF in horses were attributed to oxalate poisoning because oxalate crystals were observed in renal tubules [70,71]. Horses seem to be more resistant than other domestic species to oxalate-induced renal damage, however, and experimental administration of various forms of oxalate (in large doses) produces hypocalcemia and gastrointestinal signs rather than renal failure. Further, long-term ingestion of plants containing oxalate produces fibrous osteodystrophy (oxalates bind calcium in the intestinal tract, decreasing intestinal calcium absorption), but renal damage in affected horses has been minimal [72]. It is now recognized that formation of oxalate crystals in diseased equine kidneys is a secondary change likely related to stasis of urine in damaged renal tubules [73].

Amyloidosis is another unusual cause of CRF in horses. Systemic amyloidosis has been recognized in horses hyperimmunized for antiserum production, but hepatic and splenic involvement were more common than renal involvement in these horses [74]. Accumulation and tissue localization of amyloid exhibit considerable species variation and amyloid deposition in the kidney is most common in dogs and cattle, with renal amyloidosis remaining a significant cause of CRF in dogs [75]. Renal neoplasia is a final cause of CRF in horses but in most affected horses tumors are unilateral and produce weight loss, intermittent colic, and hematuria rather than CRF.

Clinical signs

Horses with CRF often present relatively late in the disease course, when their owners note lethargy, anorexia, and weight loss. A history of months to years of polydipsia in some cases supports renal disease of long duration. In other animals prior disease (eg, colic, colitis, or pleuropneumonia) or prolonged medication (aminoglycoside antibiotics or nonsteroidal anti-inflammatory drugs) use may provide important information about the initiation and duration of renal failure. In most cases, however, the onset is insidious and it is not possible to identify a precipitating event or determine the duration of renal disease.

Chronic weight loss is the most common presenting complaint for horses with CRF [55–57]. Partial anorexia, ventral edema, polyuria-polydipsia, rough hair coat, lethargy, and poor athletic performance are other concerns. In addition, horses with advanced CRF may have a characteristic "fishy" odor that likely reflects increased urea excretion in sweat. In the review of 99 horses with CRF weight loss, polyuria-polydipsia, and ventral edema were reported in 79 (86%) of 92, 38 (56%) of 68, and 34 (42%) of 80 cases, respectively [21]. Lethargy and weight loss can be attributed to several factors. An increase in the concentration of nitrogenous wastes in blood can have a direct central appetite-suppressant effect that can lead to partial or complete anorexia [3]. Next, as azotemia progresses, excess urea diffuses across gastrointestinal epithelium where it is metabolized to ammonia and carbon dioxide by bacterial ureases. In the oral cavity, excess ammonia can lead to excessive dental tartar formation, gingivitis, and oral ulcers. In the gastrointestinal tract, excess urea and ammonia can lead to ulceration and mild to moderate protein-losing enteropathy, and severely uremic animals may produce soft feces. The prolonged half-life of gastrin (eliminated through the kidneys) may contribute further to gastric ulcer disease because of increased acid secretion. Finally, as the combined effects of uremic toxins render the affected patient "catabolic," body mass declines as body reserves are tapped to meet basal energy requirements.

Mild ventral edema with CRF may be attributable to three factors: (1) decreased oncotic pressure; (2) increased vascular permeability; and (3) increased hydrostatic pressure (hypertension). Because albumin accounts for approximately 75% of plasma colloid oncotic pressure, decreases in albumin concentration (below about 2 g/dL) can decrease plasma oncotic pressure despite a normal total plasma protein concentration [76]. The effects of uremic toxins on endothelial cell membranes can alter vascular permeability and contribute to edema [3]. Chronic renal insufficiency can lead to renal hypoxia and hypoperfusion, which stimulate renal juxtaglomerular cells to release renin. Activation of the RAAS tends to elevate blood (and capillary hydrostatic) pressure and contribute to edema. Activation of the RAAS also leads to increased sodium reabsorption in both the proximal (direct effect of angiotensin II) and distal (effect of aldosterone) tubules. Sodium retention leads to expansion of circulating volume further contributing to edema formation. Alterations in blood pressure in horses with CRF [46] have not been routinely evaluated as they have in small animal and human patients, nor have increased circulating concentrations of angiotensin II or aldosterone been documented. The nephrotic syndrome, characterized by edema, hypoalbuminemia, and heavy proteinuria, is not as well-documented in horses compared with small animals and humans with CRF. Horses with CRF, however, seem less at risk for the significant pleural effusion or ascites that can accompany the nephrotic syndrome in small animals [1].

Polyuria-polydipsia is a variable finding in horses with CRF and the magnitude of polyuria does not seem to be correlated to the level of azotemia in clinical cases. Typically, daily urine volume may be twice that of normal horses such that many clients do not recognize polyuria, especially when horses are not housed in stalls. Variation in water intake among normal horses and common use of automatic waterers and large stock tanks also make it more difficult to recognize polydipsia. Mechanisms by which polyuria develops in patients with CRF include (1) increased tubule flow rate in surviving nephrons; (2) decreased medullary hypertonicity; and (3) impaired response of collecting ducts to vasopressin (acquired nephrogenic diabetes insipidus) [1,2].

An early complaint for horses with CRF can be poor performance. Poor performance may be related to mild anemia (packed cell volume 25%–30%) and lethargy. Although the anemia of CRF has been attributed to several factors including blood loss, decreased erythrocyte survival time, nutritional deficiencies, and decreased erythropoietin activity, the latter has clearly emerged as the principal cause of anemia in humans and small animals with CRF [1,77]. Administration of recombinant human erythropoietin to patients awaiting kidney transplant has been one of the most significant advances in management of human CRF, because it has eliminated the need for blood transfusions, improved exercise capacity, and decreased morbidity associated with the uremic syndrome [77].

Diagnosis

Although many clinical signs of CRF are nonspecific, accumulation of excess dental tartar (especially on the canine teeth) and a uremic odor are signs that should raise clinical suspicion. Owners should be specifically questioned with regard to prior medical history, medication use, and water consumption and urine output. Physical examination should include transrectal palpation of the bladder and left kidney and the course of both ureters from the bladder neck to the kidneys should be followed to determine whether they are enlarged. The left kidney may be firm with an irregular surface and ureters, usually undetectable in normal horses, may be thickened in horses with CRF and ureteroliths can occasionally be palpated.

Clinicopathologic evaluation including a complete blood count, serum chemistry profile, and urinalysis often yields results that are diagnostic for CRF. Specifically, the combination of azotemia, hypercalcemia, and persistent isosthenuria (urine-specific gravity of 1.008–1.012 or up to 1.020 with heavy proteinuria) strongly supports a diagnosis of CRF in horses. Although the magnitude of azotemia at the time of initial diagnosis may vary, most affected horses have a BUN:Cr ratio (in units of milligrams per deciliter) greater than 10:1 (whereas the BUN:Cr ratio is generally less than 10:1 with prerenal azotemia and ARF). In the series of 99 horses with CRF, further abnormal laboratory data included mild anemia (40%); albumin concentration less than 2.5 g/dL (86%); hyponatremia (65%); hyperkalemia (56%); hypochloremia (46%); hypercalcemia (67%);

and hypophosphatemia (47%) [21]. Acid-base balance is often normal, although metabolic acidosis may develop in the terminal stages of CRF.

With the exception of hypercalcemia and hypophosphatemia (Williams-Smith syndrome), electrolyte alterations in horses with CRF tend to be less severe than with ARF [78]. Hypercalcemia in horses with CRF is not a result of increased parathormone action [79]. Rather, horses absorb excessive amounts of dietary calcium across the intestinal tract and eliminate the excess as calcium carbonate (and to a lesser extent calcium oxalate) crystals in urine. In horses with CRF, urinary calcium excretion is reduced and the magnitude of hypercalcemia varies with the amount of calcium in the diet. Changing from a high-calcium diet (alfalfa) to a lower-calcium diet (pasture or grass hay) can return serum calcium concentration to within the reference range within a couple of days [55,78]. Although soft tissue mineralization has been described with hypercalcemia associated with vitamin D toxicity or the paraneoplastic syndrome, the author is unaware of clinical problems attributed to either hypercalcemia or hypophosphatemia in horses with CRF.

Failing kidneys seem to have a tremendous adaptive capacity to maintain tubular function until GFR is quite low [5]. In the author's experience, tubular dysfunction resulting in significant sodium or phosphorous wasting (manifested by increased fractional clearance values) and glucosuria is more common with ARF than with CRF. Similarly, increased urinary activity of γ-glutamyltransferase, a sensitive marker of proximal tubule damage, is rarely elevated in CRF. Isosthenuria is the main finding on urinalysis; however, gross inspection of urine samples reveals that they are notably less viscid and contain few crystals compared with normal horse urine. Increased numbers of calcium oxalate crystals may also be observed on sediment examination; however, this more likely reflects the lesser amount of calcium carbonate crystals excreted in urine of horses with CRF. Because pyelonephritis can be a cause of CRF, a quantitative urine culture should be performed during initial evaluation of horses with CRF because positive results ($> 10,000$ cfu/mL) can be obtained in the absence of obvious pyuria on sediment examination. In addition, urinary protein and Cr concentrations should be quantitatively measured to screen for GN as the cause of CRF. Normal horses have a urine protein:urine Cr ratio (both in milligrams per deciliter) that is less than 1:1 (often less than 0.1:1) [80], whereas horses with GN and significant proteinuria often have a urine protein:urine Cr ratio greater than 3:1 [2,46,53].

Transabdominal ultrasonographic imaging of the kidneys is indicated in all equids with a suspected diagnosis of CRF to determine renal size, architecture, and echogenicity [81,82]. With CRF kidneys are often small with an irregular surface and echogenicity, compared with the spleen for the left kidney, is variably increased because of renal fibrosis. Additional findings may include nephrolithiasis with or without hydronephrosis. Occasionally the renal pelvis appears hyperechoic because of accumulation of a crystalline "sludge" but the hallmark of a true nephrolith is presence of an acoustic shadow deep to the stone (Fig. 2). Renal biopsy using ultrasonographic guidance can also be performed to document renal disease. When horses are presented for evaluation in the later stages of disease, biopsy results typically reveal glomerular, tubular, and interstitial lesions consistent with ESRD. Rarely do biopsy results provide information about the inciting cause of renal disease and renal biopsy is not strongly recommended for horses with advanced disease. In contrast, renal biopsy results may be more informative in horses with mild azotemia (serum Cr concentration <5 mg/dL). Because lesions may not be homogenously distributed throughout the kidney, however, biopsy results can range from essentially normal renal tissue to extensive changes in horses with similar magnitudes of azotemia. Further, renal biopsy samples collected from people with renal disease are routinely examined by immunohistochemistry and electron microscopy in addition to light microscopy with multiple stains. Because renal biopsies collected from veterinary patients are typically examined by light

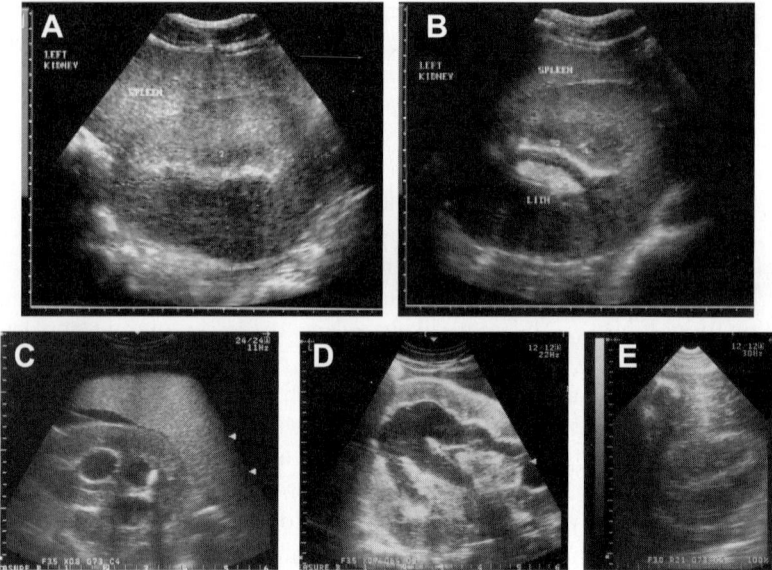

Fig. 2. Ultrasonographic images of the left kidney of two horses afflicted with chronic renal failure. (A) Left kidney of a yearling with chronic interstitial nephritis that developed 11 months following treatment with an aminoglycoside antibiotic and flunixin meglumine for a leg wound; note the generalized increase in echogenicity of the renal parenchyma in comparison to the spleen. (B) Left kidney of the same yearling with the probe aimed in a different plane revealing a large nephrolith adjacent to the renal pelvis. (C) Left kidney of a stallion with an obstructive ureterolith causing hydronephrosis; note the small nephrolith in the center of the image producing an acoustic shadow. (D) Left kidney of the same stallion imaged in a plane rotated 90o revealing hydronephrosis consequent to obstructive disease. (E) Left kidney of the same stallion following relief of ureteral obstruction by electrolhydraulic lithotripsy; note that the kidney is small and renal parenchyma has a diffuse increase in echogenicity caused by renal fibrosis.

microscopy alone, only limited information can be gleaned from this diagnostic procedure.

The severity of CRF in affected horses can be assessed by several means; the magnitude of azotemia is the most practical parameter but azotemia is insensitive until the later stages of CRF. In general, Cr concentration is a more reliable measure than BUN, and doubling of Cr roughly correlates to a 50% decline in GFR. Serum Cr concentrations in the range of 5 to 10 mg/dL indicate a marked decline in renal function, and values exceeding 15 mg/dL are consistent with a grave prognosis. In contrast, horses with a Cr concentration below 5 mg/dL may exhibit few clinical signs and can be successfully managed for months or years. Measurement of GFR provides the most accurate quantitative assessment of renal function, but it is rarely pursued because it is more time consuming and technically demanding than measurement of serum Cr concentration. Although a number of methods are available to measure GFR (see reference [2] for review), measurement of endogenous Cr clearance or the plasma disappearance of exogenously administered Cr or 99-metastable technetium tagged to diethylenetriamine pentaacetic acid are the most practical methods in a clinical setting. The former requires timed urine collections, whereas the latter requires nuclear medicine capabilities. Because baseline GFR in normal horses can range from 1.5 to 3 mL/kg/min, a single measurement of GFR in horses with CRF may be difficult to interpret. Repeated measurement of GFR in an individual, however, remains the most sensitive means to monitor progression of CRF over time [1,2].

Management

At the time of presentation most horses with CRF exhibit obvious weight loss and other clinical signs. Because of the progressive and irreversible nature of the renal disease, the long-term prognosis is grave. Renal replacement therapy (peritoneal dialysis, hemodialysis, and renal transplantation) is not available for horses with CRF. CRF consequent to pyelonephritis could be considered an exception, because antibiotic treatment could, in theory, lead to resolution of infection and improved renal function. Unfortunately, significant renal damage has usually occurred by the time the diagnosis is established in most cases of bilateral pyelonephritis and the prognosis for a return to normal renal function is guarded to poor.

The short-term prognosis for horses with CRF is more favorable. Horses with serum Cr concentrations less than 5 mg/dL may remain in fairly good condition for months to several years with minimal deterioration. In contrast, CRF patients with serum Cr concentrations greater than 10 mg/dL general do not survive for more than a few weeks, whereas those with a serum Cr concentration in the range of 5 to 10 mg/dL have variable outcomes. With lower levels of azotemia (<5 mg/dL), clinical signs of uremia are not apparent and the primary clinical problem may be polyuria-polydipsia. It is impossible to predict which patients will deteriorate more rapidly, but recent history and initial ability to counteract weight loss with improved management are useful indicators. Laboratory analysis of blood samples at 2- to 4-month intervals to follow the magnitude of azotemia and serum electrolyte alterations may be useful in monitoring disease progression. In general, animals that are eating well and maintain reasonable body condition carry the best short-term prognosis and may still be able to perform some limited work. Although use as breeding animals may be reduced, the author has managed two stallions with CRF through additional breeding seasons and one mare with CIN and a serum Cr concentration ranging from 8 to 10 mg/dL successfully carried a foal to term and produced adequate milk for the foal to be reared in a normal fashion. The goal in each case is to provide appropriate supportive care and to monitor the horse closely to be able to perform humane euthanasia before the patient develops uremic decompensation.

Once significant renal disease is established, irreversible decline in GFR and progression of renal failure generally ensue [5–8]. Management of equids with CRF involves palliative efforts to minimize further loss of renal function. The goals are to prevent complicating conditions (eg, by providing plenty of fresh water); to discontinue administration of nephrotoxic agents; and to provide a palatable diet to encourage appetite and minimize further weight loss. At the time of initial diagnosis, a short (24–48 hour) course of intravenous fluid therapy to promote diuresis, usually with 0.9% sodium chloride solution at twice the maintenance rate, may benefit patients that suffer a sudden exacerbation of CRF (acute on chronic disease). Fluid therapy can produce variable results with the level of azotemia declining more than 50% in some patients, whereas minimal changes are observed in other horses. Fluid therapy must be administered cautiously with body weight determined every 12 to 24 hours, because horses with CRF can develop volume overload and significant pulmonary and peripheral edema after administration of as little as 20 L of fluids [2]. An alternative approach that is more economic and may be less likely to produce significant edema is to administer 8 L of an isotonic saline solution by a nasogastric tube three times a day for 2 to 4 days. Finally, diuresis can be maintained by providing good-quality pasture (often <10% dry matter intake) as the primary diet for affected horses. Edema is not usually a significant problem in horses with CRF and mild edema should be tolerated (rather than treated with diuretics, which are largely ineffective or could lead to further electrolyte loss) unless it interferes with ambulation.

In the rare patient with obstructive nephrolithiasis or ureterolithiasis, stone removal may lead to improvement in renal function. Electrohydraulic or laser lithotripsy via an endoscope inserted into the ureter is the recommended approach to treatment in these cases [83]. Although nephrectomy remains the treatment of choice for treatment of unilateral upper urinary tract infection and lithiasis, this surgical procedure is contraindicated in patients with azotemia and CRF.

Substituting high-calcium and high-protein feed sources, such as alfalfa hay with good-quality grass hay and carbohydrates (corn and oats), may help control hypercalcemia and the level of azotemia, specifically BUN. Ideally, hay and grain should contain an adequate, but not excessive, amount of protein (less than 10% crude protein), which should maintain the BUN:Cr ratio at a target value of 10:1 [57]. It is important to provide unlimited access to fresh water and to encourage adequate energy intake by feeding a variety of palatable feeds, including fat supplementation. If appetite for grass hay deteriorates, it is preferable to offer less than ideal feeds, such as alfalfa hay, or increased amounts of concentrate to meet energy requirements and reduce the rate of weight loss. Often horses continue to graze at pasture when their appetite for hay is diminished and good-quality pasture is the ideal diet for horses with CRF.

The progressive renal injury that occurs in CRF is associated with continued damage to glomerular and tubular membranes mediated by ongoing activation of the inflammatory cascade [6–8]. In theory, treatment with antioxidant medications and free radical scavengers (vitamins C and E) could be of benefit, but current experimental data are inconclusive [84]. Similarly, there has been considerable interest in the role of dietary fat source as precursors of eicosanoids. Specifically, dietary supplementation with sources rich in omega-3 fatty acids (fish oils and vegetable oils rich in linolenic acid) seems to decrease generation of more damaging fatty acid metabolites during activation of the inflammatory cascade [85]. Diets supplemented with fish oil slowed the progression of both experimentally induced and spontaneously occurring CRF in dogs and cats [86–88]. At present, the potential benefits of feeding omega-3 fatty acids to horses with CRF are not known but when supplementation with dietary fat is pursued to increase caloric intake, it seems logical to select a supplement that is rich in omega-3 fatty acids.

Administration of medications to limit the intrarenal inflammatory response associated with CRF, especially GN, may attenuate further renal injury. Corticosteroids and aspirin have been used in patients with GN [46]; unfortunately, nonspecific blockade of prostaglandin production can have the negative effect of decreasing production of important renal vasodilating agents (prostaglandin E_2 and prostacyclin). These negative drug effects on renal blood flow may outweigh possible benefits, and their use is currently only recommended in managing horses with GN and substantial proteinuria (urine protein:urine Cr > 2:1).

Because proteinuria is a well-documented factor leading to progression of CRF [6–8], medical management of proteinuria has become an important aspect of managing CKD in people and small animals [89,90]. Activation of the RAAS resulting in angiotensin II production is of considerable importance, because angiotensin II is a potent constrictor of glomerular efferent arterioles [91]. Activation of the intrarenal RAAS can produce significant glomerular hypertension without producing increases in systemic angiotensin II concentration or blood pressure. Administration of angiotensin-converting enzyme inhibitors and specific angiotensin II receptor antagonists is now widely used in people and small animals with proteinuria to limit progression of CKD [89,90]. There are no reports of use of angiotensin-converting enzyme inhibitors in horses with CRF accompanied by proteinuria and expense of daily treatment limits use of these medications to select patients.

Finally, a number of investigators are currently focusing on developing therapeutic strategies that may modulate or limit renal fibrosis [92,93]. Studies of the effects of cytokines, lymphokines, and proteoglycans on matrix synthesis and degradation by mesangial cells and on fibroblast activation in damaged glomeruli may lead to novel treatment options in the future.

References

[1] Polzin DJ, Osborne CA, Bartges JW, et al. Chronic renal failure. In: Ettinger SJ, Feldman EC, editors. Textbook of veterinary internal medicine, vol. 2. 4th edition. Philadelphia: WB Saunders; 1995. p. 1734–60.

[2] Schott HC. Chronic renal failure. In: Reed SM, Bayly WM, Sellon DC, editors. Equine internal medicine. 2nd edition. Philadelphia: WB Saunders; 2004. p. 1231–53.

[3] Meyer TW, Hostetter TH. Uremia. N Engl J Med 2007;357(13):1316–25.

[4] Traub-Dargatz JL, Fettman MJ, Dargatz D. Identifying the cause of weight loss in horses. Vet Med 1992;87(4):346–56.

[5] Hayslett JP. Functional adaptation to reduction in renal mass. Physiol Rev 1979;59(1): 137–69.

[6] Hostetter TH. Progression of renal disease and renal hypertrophy. Annu Rev Physiol 1995; 57:263–78.

[7] Brown SA, Crowell WA, Brown CA, et al. Pathophysiology and management of progressive renal disease. Vet J 1997;154(2):93–109.

[8] Finco DR, Brown SA, Brown CA, et al. Progression of chronic renal disease in the dog. J Vet Intern Med 1999;13(6):516–28.

[9] Weiner DE. Causes and consequences of chronic kidney disease: implications for managed health care. J Manag Care Pharm 2007;13(Suppl 3):S1–9.

[10] Hostetter TH. Prevention of the development and progression of renal disease. J Am Soc Nephrol 2003;14:S144–7.

[11] Grauer GF. Early detection of renal damage and disease in dogs and cats. Vet Clin North Am Small Anim Pract 2005;35(3):581–96.

[12] Pugliese A, Gruppillo A, Di Pietro S. Clinical nutrition in gerontology: chronic renal disorders of the dog and cat. Vet Res Commun 2005;29(Suppl 2):57–63.

[13] Ross SJ, Osborne CJ, Kirk CA, et al. Clinical evaluation of dietary modification for treatment of spontaneous chronic kidney disease in cats. J Am Vet Med Assoc 2006;229(6): 949–57.

[14] Brosnahan MM, Paradis MR. Demographic and clinical characteristics of geriatric horses: 467 cases (1989–1999). J Am Vet Med Assoc 2003;223(1):93–8.

[15] Irwin DHG, Howell DW. Equine pyelonephritis and unilateral nephrectomy. J S Afr Vet Assoc 1980;51(4):235–6.

[16] Trotter GW, Brown CM, Ainsworth DM. Unilateral nephrectomy for treatment of a renal abscess in a foal. J Am Vet Med Assoc 1984;184(11):1392–4.

[17] Juzwiak JS, Bain FT, Slone DE, et al. Unilateral nephrectomy for treatment of chronic hematuria due to nephrolithiasis in a colt. Can Vet J 1988;29(11):931–3.

[18] Mitchell KJ, Dowling BA, Hughes KJ, et al. Unilateral nephrectomy as a treatment for renal trauma in a foal. Aust Vet J 204;82(12):753–5.

[19] Sullins KE, McIlwraith CW, Yovich JV, et al. Ectopic ureter managed by unilateral nephrectomy in two female horses. Equine Vet J 1988;20(6):463–6.

[20] Röcken M, Mosel G, Stehle C, et al. Left- and right-sided laparoscopic-assisted nephrectomy in standing horses with unilateral renal disease. Vet Surg 2007;36(6):568–72.

[21] Schott HC, Patterson KS, Fitzerald SD, et al. Chronic renal failure in 99 horses. In: Proceedings of the 43rd Annual Convention of the American Association of Equine Practitioners. 1997. p. 345–6.

[22] Andrews FM, Rosol TJ, Kohn CW, et al. Bilateral renal hypoplasia in four young horses. J Am Vet Med Assoc 1986;189(2):209–12.

[23] Anderson WI, Picut CA, King JM, et al. Renal dysplasia in a Standardbred colt. Vet Pathol 1988;25(2):179–80.

[24] Jones SL, Langer DL, Sterner-Kock A, et al. Renal dysplasia and benign ureteropelvic polyps associated with hydronephrosis in a foal. J Am Vet Med Assoc 1994;204(8): 1230–4.

[25] Zicker SC, Marty GD, Carlson GP, et al. Bilateral renal dysplasia with nephron hypoplasia in a foal. J Am Vet Med Assoc 1990;196(12):2001–5.

[26] Ramirez S, Williams J, Seahorn TL, et al. Ultrasound-assisted diagnosis of renal dysplasia in a 3-month-old Quarter Horse colt. Vet Radiol Ultrasound 1998;39(2):143–6.

[27] Gull T, Schmitz DG, Bahr A. Renal hypoplasia and dysplasia in an American miniature foal. Vet Rec 2001;149(7):199–203.

[28] Ronen N, van Amstel SR, Nesbit JW, et al. Renal dysplasia in two adult horses: clinical and pathological aspects. Vet Rec 1988;132(11):269–70.

[29] Woolridge AA, Seahorn JL, Williams J, et al. Chronic renal failure associated with nephrolithiasis, ureterolithiasis, and renal dysplasia in a 2-year-old Quarter Horse gelding. Vet Radiol Ultrasound 1999;40(4):361–4.

[30] Scott PC, Vasey J. Progressive polycystic renal disease in an aged horse. Aust Vet J 1986; 63(3):92.

[31] Ramsey G, Rothwell TLW, Gibson KT, et al. Polycystic kidneys in an adult horse. Equine Vet J 1987;19(3):243–4.

[32] Bertone JJ, Traub-Dargatz JL, Fettman MJ, et al. Monitoring the progression of renal failure in a horse with polycystic kidney disease: use of the reciprocal of serum creatinine concentration and sodium sulfanilate clearance half-time. J Am Vet Med Assoc 1987; 191(5):565–8.

[33] Aguilero-Tejero E, Estepa JC, Lopez I, et al. Polycystic kidneys as a cause of chronic renal failure and secondary hypoparathyroidism in a horse. Equine Vet J 2000;32(2):167–9.

[34] Chandler KJ, Johnston HM, Murphy DM. Polycystic kidney disease in an aged pony. Vet Rec 2003;153(24):754–6.

[35] Rizk D, Chapman AB. Cystic and inherited kidney diseases. Am J Kidney Dis 2003;42(6): 1305–17.

[36] Torres VE, Harris PC, Pirson Y. Autosomal dominant polycystic kidney disease. Lancet 2007;369(9569):1287–301.

[37] O'Leary CA, MacKay BM, Malik R, et al. Polycystic kidney disease in bull terriers: an autosomal dominant inherited disorder. Aust Vet J 1999;77(6):361–6.

[38] Biller DS, Dibartola SP, Eaton KA, et al. Inheritance of polycystic kidney disease in Persian cats. J Hered 1996;87(1):1–5.

[39] Young AE, Biller DS, Herrgessell EJ, et al. Feline polycystic kidney disease is linked to the PKD1 region. Mamm Genome 2005;16(1):59–65.

[40] Barthez PY, Rivier P, Begon D. Prevalence of polycystic kidney disease in Persian and Persian related cats in France. J Feline Med Surg 2003;5(6):345–7.

[41] O'Leary CA, Ghoddusi M, Huxtable CR. Renal pathology of polycystic kidney disease and concurrent hereditary nephritis in Bull Terriers. Aust Vet J 2002;80(6):353–61.

[42] White RH, Raafat F, Milford DV, et al. The Alport nephropathy: clinicopathological correlations. Pediatr Nephrol 2005;20(7):897–903.

[43] Okada K, Ishikawa N, Fujimori K, et al. Abnormal development of nephrons in claudin-16-defective Japanese black cattle. J Vet Med Sci 2005;67(2):171–8.

[44] Banks KL, Henson JB. Immunologically mediated glomerulitis of horses. II. Antiglomerular basement membrane antibody and other mechanisms of spontaneous disease. Lab Invest 1972;26(6):708–15.

[45] Osborne CA, Hammer RF, Stevens JB, et al. The glomerulus in health and disease: a comparative review of domestic animals and man. Adv Vet Sci Comp Med 1977;21:207–85.

[46] Van Biervliet J, Divers TJ, Porter B, et al. Glomerulonephritis in horses. Compendium on Continuing Education for the Practicing Veterinarian 2002;24(11):892–902.

[47] Banks KL, Henson JB, McGuire TC. Immunologically mediated glomerulitis of horses. I. Pathogenesis in persistent infection by equine infectious anemia virus. Lab Invest 1972; 26(6):701–7.

[48] Morter RL, Williams RD, Bolte H, et al. Equine leptospirosis. J Am Vet Med Assoc 1969; 155(2):436–42.

[49] Hogan PM, Bernard WV, Kazakevicius PA, et al. Acute renal disease due to *Leptospira interrogansa* in a weanling. Equine Vet J 1996;28(4):331–3.

[50] Frazer ML. Acute renal failure from leptospirosis in a foal. Aust Vet J 1999;77(8):499–500.

[51] Rodriguez-Iturbe B, Batsford S. Pathogenesis of poststreptococcal glomerulonephritis a century after Clemens von Pirquet. Kidney Int 2007;71(11):1094–104.

[52] Roberts MC, Kelly WR. Renal dysfunction in a case of purpura haemorrhagica in a horse. Vet Rec 1982;110(7):144–6.

[53] Divers TJ, Timoney JF, Lewis RM, et al. Equine glomerulonephritis and renal failure associated with complexes of group-C streptococcal antigen and IgG antibody. Vet Immunol Immunopathol 1992;32(1–2):93–102.

[54] McSloy A, Poulsen K, Fisher PJ. Diagnosis and treatment of a selective immunoglobulin M glomerulonephropathy in a Quarter Horse gelding. J Vet Intern Med 2007;21(4): 874–7.

[55] Tennant B, Kaneko JJ, Lowe JE, et al. Chronic renal failure in the horse. In: Proceedings of the 24th Annual Convention of the American Association of Equine Practitioners. 1978. p. 293–7.

[56] Koterba AM, Coffman JR. Acute and chronic renal disease in the horse. Compendium on Continuing Education for the Practicing Veterinarian 1981;3(12):S461–9.

[57] Divers TJ. Chronic renal failure in horses. Compendium on Continuing Education for the Practicing Veterinarian 1983;5(6):S310–7.

[58] Divers TJ, Whitlock RH, Byars TD, et al. Acute renal failure in six horses resulting from haemodynamic causes. Equine Vet J 1987;19(3):178–84.

[59] Schmitz DG. Toxic nephropathy in horses. Compendium on Continuing Education for the Practicing Veterinarian 1988;10(1):104–11.

[60] Block CA, Schoolwerth AC. The epidemiology and outcome of acute renal failure and the impact on chronic kidney disease. Semin Dial 2006;19(6):450–4.

[61] Boyd WL, Bishop LM. Pyelonephritis of horses and cattle. J Am Vet Med Assoc 1937;90: 154–62.

[62] Held JP, Wright B, Henton JE. Pyelonephritis associated with renal failure in a horse. J Am Vet Med Assoc 1986;189(6):688–9.

[63] Carrick JB, Pollitt CC. Chronic pyelonephritis in a brood mare. Aust Vet J 1987;64(8): 252–4.

[64] Sloet van Oldruitenborgh-Oosterbaan MM, Klabec HC. Ureteropyelonephritis in a Fresian mare. Vet Rec 1988;122(25):609–10.

[65] Hope WD, Wilson JH, Hager DA, et al. Chronic renal failure associated with bilateral nephroliths and ureteroliths in a two-year-old Thoroughbred colt. Equine Vet J 1989;21(3): 228–31.

[66] Ehnen SJ, Divers TJ, Gillette D, et al. Obstructive nephrolithiasis and ureterolithiasis associated with chronic renal failure in horses: eight cases (1981–1987). J Am Vet Med Assoc 1990;197(2):249–53.

[67] Divers TJ. Nephrolithiasis and ureterolithiasis in horses and their association with renal disease and failure. Equine Vet J 1989;21(3):161–2.

[68] Coe FL, Evan A, Worcester E. Kidney stone disease. J Clin Invest 2005;115(10): 2598–608.

[69] Kodner CM, Kudrimoti A. Diagnosis and management of acute interstitial nephritis. Am Fam Physician 2003;67(12):2527–34.

[70] Webb RF, Knight PR. Oxalate nephropathy in a horse. Aust Vet J 1977;53(11):554–5.

[71] Andrews EJ. Oxalate nephropathy in a horse. J Am Vet Med Assoc 1971;159(1):49–52.

[72] Walthall JC, McKenzie RA. Osteodystrophia fibrosa in horses at pasture in Queensland: field and laboratory investigations. Aust Vet J 1976;52(1):11–6.

[73] Roberts MC, Seiler RJ. Renal failure in a horse with chronic glomerulonephritis and renal oxalosis. J Equine Med Surg 1979;3(6):278–83.

[74] Jakob W. Spontaneous amyloidosis of animals. Vet Pathol 1971;8:292–306.

[75] Cook AK, Cowgill LD. Clinical and pathological features of protein-losing glomerular disease in the dog: a review of 137 cases (1985–1992). J Am Anim Hosp Assoc 1996;32(4): 313–22.

[76] Pearson EG. Hypoalbuminemia in horses. Compend Contin Educ Pract Vet 1990;12(4): 555–60.

[77] Robinson BE. Epidemiology of chronic kidney disease and anemia. J Am Med Dir Assoc 2006;7(Suppl 9):S3–6.

[78] Tennant B, Bettleheim P, Kaneko JJ. Paradoxic hypercalcemia and hypophosphotemia associated with chronic renal failure in horses. J Am Vet Med Assoc 1982;180(6):630–4.

[79] Brobst DF, Bayly WM, Reed SM, et al. Parathyroid hormone evaluation in normal horses and horses with renal failure. J Equine Vet Sci 1982;2(5):150–7.

[80] Kohn CW, Strasser SL. 24-hour renal clearance and excretion of endogenous substances in the mare. Am J Vet Res 1986;47(6):1332–7.

[81] Hoffmann KL, Wood AK, McCarthy PH. Sonographic-anatomic correlation and imaging protocol for the kidneys of horses. Am J Vet Res 1995;56(11):1403–12.

[82] Divers TJ, Yeager AE. The value of ultrasonographic examination in the diagnosis and management of renal disease in horses. Equine Vet Educ 1995;7(6):334–41.

[83] Rodger LD, Carlson GP, Moran ME, et al. Resolution of a left ureteral stone using electrohydraulic lithotripsy in a Thoroughbred colt. J Vet Intern Med 1995;9(2):280–2.

[84] Locatelli F, Canaud B, Eckardt KU, et al. Oxidative stress in end-stage renal disease: an emerging threat to patient outcome. Nephrol Dial Transplant 2003;18(7):1272–80.

[85] Schmitz PG, Antony KA. Omega-3 fatty acids in ESRD: should patients with ESRD eat more fish? Nephrol Dial Transplant 2002;17(1):11–4.

[86] Brown SA, Brown CA, Crowell WA. Effects of dietary polyunsaturated fatty acid supplementation in early renal insufficiency in dogs. J Lab Clin Med 2000;135(3):275–86.

[87] Jacob F, Polzin DJ, Osborne CA, et al. Clinical evaluation of dietary modification for treatment of spontaneous chronic renal failure in dogs. J Am Vet Med Assoc 2002;220(8): 1163–70.

[88] Plantinga EA, Everts H, Kastelein AM, et al. Retrospective study of the survival of cats with acquired chronic renal insufficiency offered different commercial diets. J Am Vet Med Assoc 2005;157(7):185–7.

[89] Palmer BF. Proteinuria as a therapeutic target in patients with chronic kidney disease. Am J Nephrol 2007;27(3):287–93.

[90] Lefebvre HP, Brown SA, Chetboul V, et al. Angiotensin-converting enzyme inhibitors in veterinary medicine. Curr Pharm Des 2007;13(13):1347–61.

[91] Yoshioka T, Mitarai T, Kon V, et al. Role for angiotensin II in an overt functional proteinuria. Kidney Int 1986;30(4):538–45.

[92] Rodriguez-Iturbe B, Johnson RJ, Herrera-Acosta J. Tubulointerstitial damage and progres-
     sion of renal failure. Kidney Int Suppl 2005;99:S82–6.
[93] Tamada S, Asai T, Kuwabara N, et al. Molecular mechanisms and therapeutic strategies of
     chronic renal injury: the role of nuclear factor kappaB activation in the development of renal
     fibrosis. J Pharmacol Sci 2006;100(1):17–21.

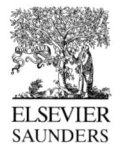

ELSEVIER
SAUNDERS

VETERINARY
CLINICS
Equine Practice

Vet Clin Equine 23 (2007) 613–629

Equine Urolithiasis

Katja F. Duesterdieck-Zellmer, DrMedVet, MS, PhD

Department of Clinical Sciences, College of Veterinary Medicine, Oregon State University,
Corvallis, OR 97331, USA

The presence of macroscopic concretions of urine crystals within the urinary tract is termed *urolithiasis*. The prevalence of equine urolithiasis has been estimated to be low: 0.04% to 0.5% of accessions or diagnoses in different equine clinics [1–3] or 0.7% in slaughtered horses in Spain [4]. In the latter population, uroliths were more commonly found in the kidneys and urinary bladder than in the ureters or urethra. In horses with clinical signs of urolithiasis, uroliths are most commonly encountered in the urinary bladder [1,5], followed by the urethra [1]. Renal or ureteral calculi are found less frequently with clinical urolithiasis, but it is not uncommon to detect uroliths in more than one location [1,5–8]. Male horses are presented more often with clinical signs of urolithiasis than mares [1,5], with geldings seeming to be more predisposed than stallions [1]. The greater prevalence in male horses is attributed to the shorter and more distensible urethra in mares, allowing them to void most uroliths before recognition of clinical signs [9,10]. It is unknown whether or not the predisposition of geldings compared with stallions is the result of a smaller urethral diameter because of castration, as has been reported in cattle [1,11].

Composition of equine calculi

Uroliths are composed of inorganic crystalloid components and smaller quantities of organic matrix [12]. Crystalloid components are described by their chemical constituents and their crystal structure. In horses, the main crystalloid component of uroliths is calcium carbonate ($CaCO_3$) [1,4–7, 13–21] in the form of calcite, the most stable hexagonal crystal form. Other forms of $CaCO_3$, such as vaterite (a metastable hexagonal crystal form) and aragonite (an orthorhombic crystal form), have also been found in equine uroliths [4,7,13–16,19]. Inorganic components contained to a lesser degree

E-mail address: katja.zellmer@oregonstate.edu

in equine urinary calculi are struvite (magnesium ammonium phosphate hexahydrate), calcium oxalate, and calcium sulfate in addition to elemental phosphorous and magnesium [1,4,6,17–19,22]. In one report, a urolith composed mostly of calcium phosphate was found [7]. Most equine uroliths are spheroid in shape and have an irregular and spiculated surface (Fig. 1), although some can be more variable in shape with a smooth surface [4,10,13,18,20,23].

The organic matrix of equine uroliths has not been examined in detail. Organic substances, primarily mucoproteins [12], identified in human uroliths include matrix substance A, Tamm-Horsfall mucoprotein, uromucoid, serum albumin, and α- and γ-globulins [24,25]. It seems that certain mucoproteins are associated with certain uroliths; for example, Tamm-Horsfall mucoprotein is commonly associated with calcium oxalate calculi in human beings [26].

In one study [1], 63% of samples collected from the center of equine uroliths were positive for bacterial growth. *Escherichia coli*, *Staphylococcus* spp, and *Streptococcus* spp were the most common isolates. Interestingly, *E coli* isolates were most often recovered from uroliths removed from male horses, whereas *Streptococcus* spp isolates were more frequently recovered from uroliths removed from female horses. No explanation for this difference was advanced by the authors of that report. Another study also found *E coli* and *Streptococcus* spp as the most common isolates from cystic calculi [21]. It warrants mention that bacterial culture of urine may yield negative results, although bacteria, often multiple isolates, can still be recovered from the urolith. Thus, attempts to assess for concurrent urinary tract infection in horses with urolithiasis should include bacterial culture of appropriately collected urine and the urolith itself (by submitting the entire urolith or fragments removed during surgery).

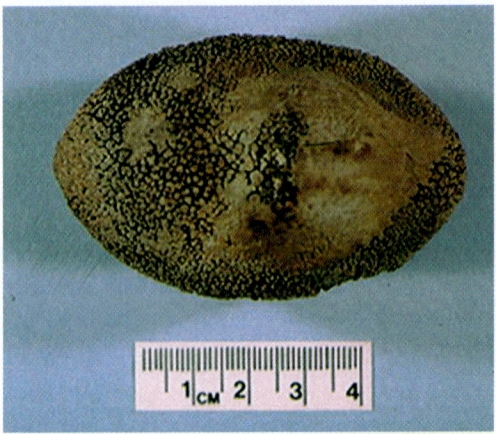

Fig. 1. Equine cystic calculus. (*Courtesy of* R.D. Howard, Gilbert, AZ.)

Pathophysiology

It is well known that horses excrete large amounts of $CaCO_3$ crystals in their urine [10,27] and that their urine pH is alkaline [28], allowing for calcite crystal formation. Urine crystals in equine urine can be recognized grossly because they contribute to the turbidity of normal equine urine. Further, a large amount of sediment can be appreciated within a few minutes after placing a sample of equine urine into a specimen container. When a microscopic sediment examination of urine is performed, these normal crystals are primarily $CaCO_3$ that appear as round to spheroid crystals of varying size; however, birefringent calcium oxalate crystals can also be found to a lesser extent on sediment examination. Because mineral supersaturation is considered the primary risk factor for urolith formation in other species [29], it is somewhat surprising that urolithiasis is not more common in horses [1]. It is also well recognized that equine urine is viscid because of the large amount of mucus secreted from glands in the renal pelves and ureters. The presence of mucus further contributes to turbidity and may inhibit aggregation of $CaCO_3$ crystals into larger uroliths. Other urine constituents and urine flow rate likely play additional roles in limiting crystal formation and growth into macroscopic urinary calculi [29,30].

Relatively little is known about formation of urinary calculi in horses; however, as in other species, mineralization around a nidus under conditions favoring crystal growth (ie, supersaturation of urine) is thought to be the inciting cause [31]. In support, nonabsorbable braided suture material in the bladder lumen has served as a nidus for urolith formation in 2 horses [1], and a piece of string served as a nidus for a cystic calculus in another horse [32]. Desquamated epithelial cells may provide a nidus in animals with urinary tract disease, but such a nidus may be difficult to detect [30] in the center of urinary calculi of horses [4,13]. It is also likely that damage to renal medulla as a result of use of nonsteroidal anti-inflammatory drugs and irritation of the mucosa of the lower tract with urinary tract infection can provide a scaffold for urolith formation [7,17,33].

Subsequent enlargement of urinary calculi proceeds by aggregation of microscopic $CaCO_3$ crystals in the form of spherules to the surface of the stone [13]. A second means of urolith growth is precipitation of crystals as cement onto the surface of the calculus. It is likely that both processes occur during the formation of equine uroliths, which is reflected by the presence of spherules embedded in cement bands in scanning electron micrographs of cut surfaces of equine uroliths (Fig. 2) [13].

Ultrastructural examination of equine uroliths has also provided evidence that crystal dissolution occurs concurrently with crystal aggregation and precipitation during growth of equine uroliths [13]. Areas of the stones that were more susceptible to dissolution seemed to contain higher amounts of magnesium, possibly because of the fact that calcite high in magnesium is more soluble than calcite with a low magnesium content [13]. The concomitant processes of aggregation and precipitation of crystals and dissolution of other areas of the developing urolith may explain why many equine uroliths have a spiculated surface and why they are often relatively easy to fragment with a lithotripter.

All uroliths contain an organic matrix in addition to the crystalloid minerals, and this matrix, primarily proteins, can influence the development of the calculus, be it negatively or positively. The influence of certain proteins on the growth of uroliths is an active area of research in human medicine, but few macromolecules have conclusively been shown to support or inhibit urolith formation in vivo, and it is possible that a protein could act as a promoter and an inhibitor of calculus growth [34]. For example, macromolecules could change the surface properties of crystals by binding to them, interfering with or promoting crystal aggregation and stone growth. Proteins that are suspected to have an inhibitory effect on calcium oxalate urolith formation and growth in people include osteopontin [29], Tamm-Horsfall glycoprotein [29,34], nephrocalcin [35], heparin [36,37], and sodium pentosan polysulfate [38].

Clinical signs of urolithiasis are absent as long as crystals and small uroliths are continuously removed from the urinary tract by means of urine flow. Uroliths that eventually cause clinical signs may be formed fixed to the urinary epithelium [34], where they have enough time to grow while being bathed in supersaturated urine [30]. Once they break free, they may be passed if their size permits or they may cause partial or total obstruction of the upper urinary tract or the urethra. Finally, they may become trapped in the urinary bladder, allowing them to increase in size over time, eventually causing clinical signs of cystic calculi.

Clinical signs and diagnosis

Clinical signs with cystic calculi include dysuria, tenesmus, hematuria (microscopic or macroscopic, often worse after exercise), and urine scalding of the hind limbs or perineum in mares because of incontinence [1,5,6,10,18,21,23,39,40]. In contrast, weight loss is the most common complaint in horses with nephroliths, most likely a consequence of chronic renal failure [1]. Signs of colic can also be seen in horses with urethral or renal calculi [1,5,10,19]. Male horses with colic signs attributable to bladder distention from an obstructive urethrolith frequently have their penis partially dropped and may repeatedly posture to urinate, although these are uncommon signs with colic pain attributable to distention of the bowel. Less frequently reported signs for urolithiasis include reluctance to exercise, stiffness of the hindquarters, or penile protrusion from the sheath [5,10,23].

Uroperitoneum may develop if rupture of the intra-abdominal portion of the urinary tract (urinary bladder or, less frequently, renal perforation) occurs [1,8,19] and was a common complication attributable to compromise of the urinary bladder in a series of five horses with urethral calculi [10].

Serum biochemical abnormalities consistent with compromised renal function are most commonly noted in horses with renal or ureteral uroliths [1,6]. On urinalysis, proteinuria, microscopic hematuria, and pyuria can be found, especially in animals with cystic or urethral calculi [1,39].

Horses with renal or ureteral calculi often have chronic renal failure, but upper tract uroliths can also be incidental necropsy findings as long as sufficient renal functional mass remains. Chronic renal failure has been reported in association with unilateral nephrolithiasis, ureterolithiasis and contralateral renal dysplasia [41], unilateral nephrolithiasis and ureterolithiasis [7], and bilateral nephrolithiasis and ureterolithiasis [6,17,42,43]. Some investigators have speculated that chronic pyelonephritis or medullary necrosis consequent to use of nonsteroidal anti-inflammatory drugs may provide a nidus for urolith formation in the upper urinary tract. Upper tract stones may or may not cause obstruction of urine flow. Detection of hydronephrosis and hydroureter on ultrasonographic imaging are supportive of obstructive disease and that the uroliths are contributing to renal failure [6,7,17]. Most nephroliths seem to be nonobstructive, however, and their presence supports chronic renal disease rather than acute renal failure in horses with azotemia [6,7].

Cystic calculi are most commonly diagnosed by rectal palpation (42 of 47 cases in one study) [1,6,18,21,23,39,40]. Transrectal ultrasonography (Fig. 3), cystoscopy (Fig. 4) [32], and scanning electron microscopy (see Fig. 2) are additional diagnostic aids. When performing a rectal examination, it is important to recognize that cystoliths are commonly found within the pelvic canal in the neck of a small bladder. Thus, they can usually be palpated with the

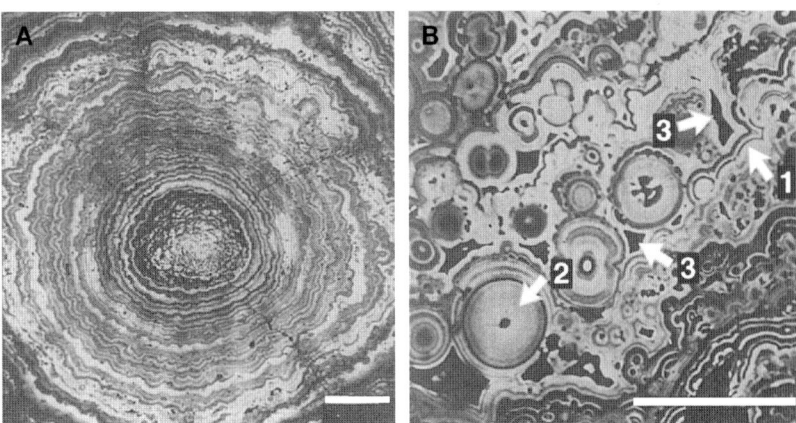

Fig. 2. Scanning electron microscopic appearance of the cut surface of equine cystic calculi. (*A*) Lower power micrograph reveals the intricate pattern of concentric banding around the core (bar = 500 μm). (*B*) Higher power micrograph reveals the ultrastructural features, including bands (1), spherules (2), and primary porosity in black (3) (bar = 50 μm). (*From* Neumann RD, Ruby AL, Ling GV, et al. Ultrastructure and mineral composition of urinary calculi from horses. Am J Vet Res 1994;55:1357; with permission.)

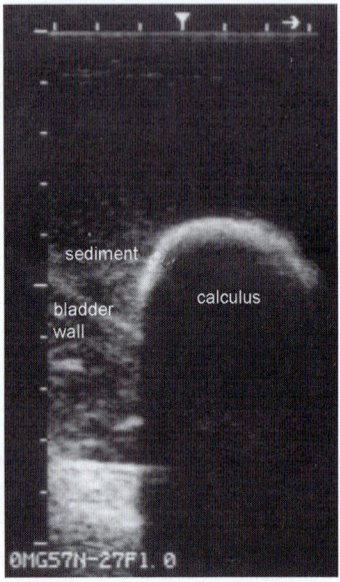

Fig. 3. Transrectal ultrasound image of a cystic calculus using a 5.5-MHz probe.

hand inserted no further than wrist deep into the rectum and can be missed if the examination is focused on structures beyond the pelvic brim. Renal and ureteral calculi are often more difficult to diagnose, but abnormal rectal palpation of the kidney [7,17,41,43] or dilation of the ureter can sometimes be detected by means of rectal palpation [6,7,41–43]. Fortunately, transabdominal and transrectal ultrasonographic imaging have substantially improved

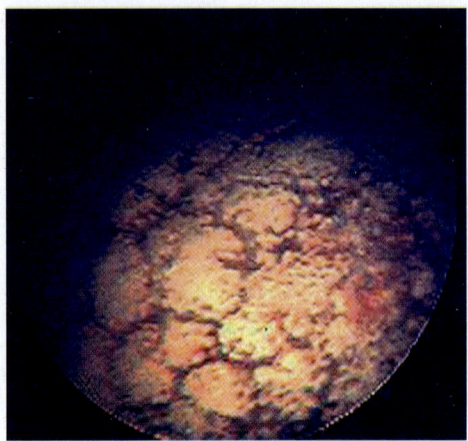

Fig. 4. Endoscopic appearance of an equine cystic calculus. (*Courtesy of* R.D. Howard, Gilbert, AZ.)

antemortem diagnosis of urolithiasis of the kidneys or ureters [7,42,44,45]. Obstructive urethral calculi can often be detected by observing urethral distention below the anus and percutaneous palpation of a stone within the urethral lumen [1,8,10]. In the single large retrospective study of horses with urolithiasis, 9% of horses had calculi in more than one location, underscoring the importance of thoroughly examining the entire urinary tract in all patients that have urolithiasis [1].

Surgical management

Numerous surgical techniques and approaches have been described for the treatment of cystic and urethral calculi in horses [1,5,10] and for the treatment of nephroliths or ureteroliths [7,44,46–49]. Surgery of the upper urinary tract can be technically challenging because of the limited exposure, especially in adult horses. Although some nephroliths and ureteroliths may spontaneously pass into the lower tract, attempts to move distal ureteral calculi into the urinary bladder by manual manipulation during laparotomy have largely been unsuccessful [43]. No matter which surgical approach is selected, the goal of surgery should be to remove all calculi from the urinary tract, with the exception of nonobstructive nephroliths. Accomplishing this goal should decrease the chance of recurrence, because small calculi or concretions remaining within the urinary tract can act as a nidus for future urolith growth [1,30]. Renal function should also be investigated before surgical intervention to remove nephroliths and ureteroliths, because signs of chronic renal failure may not resolve despite removal of the uroliths [31].

Nephrotomy

Nephrotomy is technically more difficult compared with nephrectomy because of limited surgical exposure and frequent hemorrhage from the penetrating capsular vessels [49]. One case report describes surgical removal of several nephroliths and proximal ureteroliths in a horse by means of nephrotomy; however, the horse was ultimately euthanized because of persistent signs of chronic renal failure [7].

Nephrostomy

Percutaneous nephrostomy has been described to improve renal function temporarily in a mare with bilateral obstructive ureterolithiasis [42]. A 10-French nephrostomy catheter was placed into the right renal pelvis under ultrasonographic guidance, using a guidewire and a series of dilators. After dilation of the renal pelvis with sterile saline, a 24-French thoracic catheter was placed into the renal pelvis, also under ultrasonographic guidance. The smaller catheter was used to flush the renal pelvis, whereas the larger bore catheter was used to drain the renal pelvis of urine and saline. Azotemia had improved 6 days after surgery, but the horse had to be euthanized after a cecal rupture.

Nephrectomy

Unilateral nephrectomy is usually performed in lateral recumbency through a 16th or 17th rib resection (right nephrectomy) or through a 17th or 18th rib resection (left nephrectomy) [46,49]. This procedure may be performed after a brief ventral midline exploratory laparotomy to assess both kidneys, as described in a foal [46]. Removal of the right or left kidney in foals is also feasible by means of a ventral midline approach [47,50]. Complications of this surgery include hemorrhage and adhesion formation.

The introduction of laparoscopic surgical techniques has improved surgical exposure and eliminated the need for rib resection to perform a nephrectomy [51]. Development of a hand-assisted laparoscopic technique for left nephrectomy has decreased the technical difficulty of this surgery, although uncontrollable bleeding from an accessory branch of the renal artery occurred in one of eight experimental horses [48].

Ureterorotomy

Surgical exposure of the caudal ureter is difficult in adult horses, but removal of three uroliths located within the left ureter through a left flank incision has been described [42]. The midsection of the left ureter was exposed by exteriorizing the large colon, cecum, small intestine, and cranial portion of the small colon through an additional ventral midline incision. Renal function did not improve after surgery in this horse, however [42].

Laparocystotomy

Most surgeons consider laparocystotomy the method of choice to remove cystic calculi, but poor exposure and abdominal incisional dehiscence are reported complications [1]. Approaches include caudal ventral midline [52], caudal paramedian [5,18,23], and parainguinal [40] incisions. The parainguinal approach eliminates the need for tedious dissection and ligation of branches of the external pudendal and caudal superficial epigastric vessels and the need to reflect the prepuce in male horses, creating less dead space [40]. Regardless of the approach, steady traction for several minutes is required to bring the bladder to the incision [40] and intraoperative transrectal manipulation of the calculus may facilitate removal of the stone. Subsequent closure of the cystotomy can also be challenging [5].

Laparoscopic cystotomy

Laparoscopic cystotomy provides better visualization of the urinary bladder compared with conventional laparocystotomy, permits tension-free manipulation of the bladder, and allows extraction of the cystic calculus by means of a small umbilical incision [53]. The cost of the specialized equipment is high, however, and experience in closure of the urinary bladder using laparoscopic suturing techniques is essential.

A laparoscopic technique with extra-abdominal extraction of the cystic calculus and closure of the urinary bladder has also been described [21]. This technique simplifies the bladder closure, because prior experience in laparoscopic suturing techniques is not required. It may also decrease the risk for urine leakage into the abdomen. Compared with the parainguinal laparocystotomy, the size of the incision is generally smaller.

Urethrotomy

In most mares, cystic calculi can be removed through the distensible urethral sphincter without sphincterotomy or fragmentation of the stone [1,5]. The spiculated surface of bladder stones often produces considerable trauma to the mucosa of the bladder neck and urethra, however. Thus, it can be helpful and less traumatic to manipulate the cystolith into a sterile plastic bag or surgical glove before removal from the bladder. Large stones may need to be fragmented with a manual lithotriptor or a laser device before removal and vigorous bladder lavage is subsequently used to remove the remaining small fragments. Laceration of the urethral sphincter during extraction of the urolith can be a complication when sphincterotomy is not performed, but small urethrovaginal fistulas and pollakiuria are complications described after extraction with sphincterotomy [1].

In male horses, a perineal urethrotomy can be performed in the standing position and can be a less expensive approach for removal of smaller cystic calculi. A perineal urethrotomy below the anus is also the method of choice for removal of obstructive urethral calculi [1,5,8,10,32,39], whereas a more distal urethrotomy directly over the calculus may be required for removal of urethroliths in the more distal part of the urethra [1,10]. Whelping forceps can be used to grasp cystic calculi and extract them from the urinary bladder [39], and thyroid forceps have been used to grasp urethral calculi [8]. Complications associated with the removal of a urolith through a perineal urethrotomy include rectal tear from manipulation of the stone per rectum, perforation of the bladder or pelvic urethra proximal to the urethrotomy, septic orchitis, mild peritonitis, and postoperative urethritis with tenesmus and dysuria [1,10]. In cases in which the perineal urethrotomy was left to heal by second intention, local urethral distention was most commonly noted in the area of the perineal urethrotomy and was not associated with any clinical problems [1]. Stricture of the urethra at the urethrotomy site resulting in dysuria has also been reported [5,10].

Pararectal cystotomy

This approach to the urinary bladder (also called Gökel's operation) is not commonly pursued and has a similar advantage of lower cost, as compared with laparocystotomy or laparoscopic cystotomy, for removal of cystic calculi [20,31]. The approach provides limited visual and surgical exposure of the bladder, making it a less favorable approach for most surgeons [54]. Postoperative complications can include pain on defecation, pelvic abscesses, septic peritonitis, or uroperitoneum [31,54].

Fragmentation of uroliths

Fragmentation or lithotripsy of a urinary calculus allows the removal of fragments through a smaller lumen or incision and is generally used for extraction of cystic calculi through the urethra in mares [5] or by means of a perineal urethrotomy incision in male horses. Instruments used for manual crushing include Lane bone holding or Liston bone cutting forceps [5]. In one study, however, manual crushing was associated with a high rate of recurrence (47%), likely because of incomplete removal of fragments, and 19% morbidity [1], mostly as a result of trauma to the urethra. Thus, other means of stone fragmentation should be used whenever possible.

Laser lithotripsy represents a means to fragment uroliths with less morbidity (Fig. 5). Two different lasers have been used for lithotripsy of equine uroliths: a pulsed dye laser with a wavelength of 504 nm [55,56] and a holmium: yttrium-aluminum-garnet (YAG) laser with a wavelength of 2100 nm [56–58]. The pulsed dye laser has been successful for reliable and safe lithotripsy in human patients and causes disruption of the calculus by photoacoustic effect; the laser beam creates a rapidly expanding cloud of electrons on the surface of the calculus that generates an acoustic wave greater than the tensile strength of the crystals in the urolith [55]. In contrast, the holmium:YAG laser uses photothermal (local evaporation of calculus material) and photoacoustic

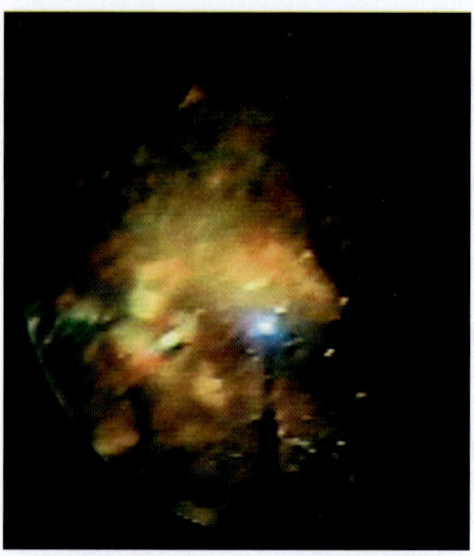

Fig. 5. Endoscopic view of laser lithotripsy of an equine cystic calculus using the pulsed dye laser lithotripter. (*Courtesy of* R.D. Howard, Gilbert, AZ.)

effects to fragment uroliths [56,57]. Cystic calculi are usually fragmented through a perineal urethrotomy incision under visual guidance with a flexible endoscope. The laser energy is delivered with an optical quartz fiber passed through the biopsy channel. It seems that the pulsed dye laser is more efficient in fragmenting large cystic calculi compared with the holmium:YAG laser; surgery times and total time of laser activation were less for the pulsed dye laser compared with the holmium:YAG laser [55–58], and the holmium:YAG laser failed to fragment 2 cystic calculi in one report [56]. Although laser lithotripsy is the treatment of choice for ureteroliths in human medicine [59], the limited availability of the pulsed dye laser, the time needed to arrange for a laser, and the costs associated with equipment rental have precluded laser lithotripsy from being more commonly used as a treatment for urolithiasis in horses.

The introduction of shock wave lithotripsy revolutionized the surgical treatment of urolithiasis in human medicine [60]. Highly focused shock waves are generated using electrohydraulic, electromagnetic, or piezoelectric devices and are aimed at the urolith. Fragmentation occurs through tensile stresses, pulverizing the calculus material, and cavitational forces [59].

Shock wave lithotripsy can be used in conjunction with a rigid cystoscope [61] or ureteroscope inserted into the urinary tract by way of the external urethral orifice or percutaneously [59]. This application is also called electrohydraulic lithotripsy, because a spark is generated by an electrode in direct contact with the calculus. The spark creates a small gas bubble that generates a shock wave that is absorbed by the calculus, resulting in shear forces that disrupt the calculus [61,62]. The disadvantage of this method of fragmentation is the cost of the equipment and experience needed to fragment the urolith expediently [61]. Several case reports of electrohydraulic lithotripsy of urinary calculi in horses exist, including the fragmentation of a left-sided ureterolith [33] and cystic calculi 5 to 8 cm in diameter [62,63]. Fragmentation was performed under general anesthesia in all cases.

Extracorporeal shock wave lithotripsy takes the technology even further by generating the shock waves outside the body and then focusing them on the urolith. This allows minimally invasive disruption of such calculi as ureteroliths or nephroliths. Complication rates are low [60], but liberation of bacteria from the urolith and obstructive urolithiasis attributable to larger fragments can occur [59]. Serious injury to adjacent tissues or organs can be caused by stray shock waves encountering an abrupt change in acoustic impedance [60]. To the author's knowledge, extracorporeal shockwave lithotripsy has not been attempted in the horse, but it has been used successfully in dogs [61].

Ballistic shock wave treatment has been used to fragment a cystic calculus approximately 8 cm in diameter in a gelding. During ballistic shock wave lithotripsy, a rigid probe is "fired" at the urolith, transferring mechanical energy to the calculus. The excursion of the probe is restricted to 2 mm, decreasing the chance of injury to the bladder wall [64]. This method of lithotripsy has been evaluated to be safe and successful for a multitude of uroliths in people; however, propulsion of fragments needing to be broken down further may be challenging during lithotripsy [65,66].

Prognosis

In one study [1], 25 (37%) of 68 horses with urolithiasis were euthanized on admission or during hospitalization. The prognosis depends on the location of the uroliths and on concurrent uroperitoneum [10] or chronic renal failure, however. Horses with renal or ureteral calculi accompanying chronic renal failure have a poor prognosis [7,17,41].

Recurrence of urolithiasis seems to be common (12 of 29 horses, recurrence within 1–32 months) but may be related to incomplete removal of all fragments from the urinary tract [1].

Prevention

$CaCO_3$ crystals form in alkaline solutions and should dissolve in acidic environments [67]. Acidification of equine urine by means of oral supplementation of ammonium chloride or ammonium sulfate has been reported to prevent recurrence of cystic calculi in a gelding with a history of recurrence of cystic calculi. Ammonium sulfate (175 mg/kg administered orally twice daily continued for 7 months) decreased urine pH to a greater extent (pH = 5.0 within 12 hours of first dose) than ammonium chloride (100 mg/kg administered orally twice daily; lowest pH = 6.5) [67]. Other investigators have reported the use of oral supplementation of ammonium chloride [2,39,63,67,68], but urine pH did not decrease reliably to less than 6.0 in all horses. In one case, ammonium chloride (40 mg/kg administered orally twice daily) was reported to cause hypersalivation and anorexia without lowering the urine pH [33]. Ascorbic acid [28] (4g administered orally twice a day [56]) has been suggested as a more palatable urinary acidifier for horses.

In human patients, increased fluid intake is the first line of therapy in the medical management of urolithiasis cases [69]. This is certainly more difficult to achieve in horses, but increasing the salt intake may result in increased water intake in horses [70].

Dietary modifications designed to reduce the intake of protein, calcium, phosphorous, and magnesium to levels recommended by the National Research Council have failed to be effective in the prevention of recurrence of urolithiasis in one horse [67]. The author does not have knowledge of any controlled studies investigating the effect of dietary protein, calcium, phosphorous, or magnesium intake on urolithiasis, however. Thus, dietary modifications aimed at decreasing protein, calcium, phosphorous, and magnesium are typically implemented after the successful resolution of urolithiasis in horses. Specifically, forage diet is changed from hays with a high calcium content (eg, alfalfa, clover) to grass hay, which has a lower calcium content.

Sabulous urolithiasis

Sabulous urolithiasis is the term used to describe the presence of sandy or gritty macroscopic concretions within the urinary bladder as a consequence of detrusor dysfunction (see the article by McKenzie elsewhere in this issue). The incidence in a population of slaughtered horses was also higher (nearly 7%) [71,72] than that of discrete urolithiasis (0.7%) [4]. It is thought that the accumulation of sabulous material within the urinary bladder is secondary to incomplete emptying of the bladder [73]. This theory has been supported by a case series of ataxia, bladder paralysis, and cystitis in horses after ingestion of *Sorghum* species [73] and a report of 3 horses with sabulous urolithiasis [5]. In the latter report, the urinary bladder was grossly distended in all horses, supporting a neurologic component to this condition. Two horses were incontinent, and one horse showed signs of dysuria. A postmortem examination of the latter horse revealed neuritis of the cauda equina, further substantiating a neurologic component of the pathophysiology of sabulous urolithiasis.

Sabulous deposits from the urinary tract of horses are mostly composed of $CaCO_3$ in the form of calcite and vaterite, with calcium oxalate, calcium phosphate, calcium sulfate, silica, magnesium, and potassium being found less frequently [71,72].

Summary

The prevalence of equine urolithiasis seems to be low. In horses with clinical signs of urolithiasis, uroliths are most commonly encountered in the urinary bladder, but it is not uncommon to detect uroliths in more than one location. The main crystalloid component of uroliths has been determined to be almost exclusively $CaCO_3$. Mineral supersaturation of urine is the driving force for mineralization of a nidus, possibly provided by desquamated cells or other organic material within the urinary tract. The most common clinical signs for cystic calculi are urine scalding of the hind limbs, hematuria, tenesmus, and dysuria. In contrast, weight loss was the most common complaint in horses with renal uroliths.

Numerous surgical techniques and approaches have been described for treatment of urolithiasis in horses. No matter which approach is chosen, the goal should be to remove all calculi completely from the urinary tract, thus decreasing the chance of recurrence of urolithiasis. The extent of renal damage and remaining renal function should be investigated before surgical intervention in horses with chronic renal failure, because the long-term prognosis with chronic renal failure is poor. Fragmentation of urinary calculi allows the removal of the fragments through a smaller incision, usually through the urethra in mares or a perineal urethrotomy in male horses. Laser and shock wave lithotripsy represent means to fragment uroliths with low morbidity.

The prognosis for horses with urolithiasis depends on the location of the urolith(s) and the degree of renal damage incurred. Recurrence of urolithiasis seems to be common but may be related to incomplete removal of all fragments from the urinary tract.

Acidification of equine urine by means of oral supplementation of ammonium chloride, ammonium sulfate, or ascorbic acid is recommended as an adjunctive therapy after surgery, as are dietary modifications aimed at increasing water intake and decreasing protein, calcium, phosphorous, and magnesium intake.

References

[1] Laverty S, Pasoce JR, Ling GV, et al. Urolithiasis in 68 horses. Vet Surg 1992;21(1):56–62.
[2] DeBowes RM, Nyrop KA, Boulton CH. Cystic calculi in the horse. Compendium of Continuing Education for the Practicing Veterinarian 1984;6(5):S268–73.
[3] Wright JG, Neal PA. Laparo-cystostomy for urinary calculus in a gelding. Vet Rec 1960; 72(8):301–3.
[4] Diaz-Espineira M, Escolar E, Bellanato J, et al. Structure and composition of equine uroliths. J Equine Vet Sci 1995;15(1):27–34.
[5] Holt PE, Pearson H. Urolithiasis in the horse—a review of 13 cases. Equine Vet J 1984;16(1): 31–4.
[6] Laing JA, Raisins AL, Rawlinson RJ, et al. Chronic renal failure and urolithiasis in a 2-year-old colt. Aust Vet J 1992;69(8):199–200.
[7] Ehnen SJ, Divers TJ, Gillette D, et al. Obstructive nephrolithiasis and ureterolithiasis associated with chronic renal failure in horses. J Am Vet Med Assoc 1990;197(2):249–53.
[8] Saam D. Urethrolithiasis and nephrolithiasis in a horse. Can Vet J 2001;42(11):880–3.
[9] Lowe JE. Surgical removal of equine uroliths via the laparocystotomy approach. J Am Vet Med Assoc 1961;139(3):345–7.
[10] Trotter GW, Bennett DG, Behm RJ. Urethral calculi in five horses. Vet Surg 1981;10(4): 159–62.
[11] Bailey CB. Siliceous urinary calculi in bulls, steers and partial castrates. Can J Anim Sci 1975; 55(2):187–91.
[12] Osborne CA, Clinton CW. Urolithiasis. Terms and concepts. Vet Clin North Am Small Anim Pract 1986;16(1):3–17.
[13] Neumann RD, Ruby AL, Ling GV, et al. Ultrastructure and mineral composition of urinary calculi from horses. Am J Vet Res 1994;55(10):1357–67.
[14] Sutor DJ, Wooley SE. Animal calculi: an X-ray diffraction study of their crystalline composition. Res Vet Sci 1970;11(3):299–301.
[15] Grünberg W. Karbonat-Harnsteine herbivorer Säugetiere. Zentralbl Veterinarmed A 1971; 18(9):767–96 [in German].
[16] Mair TS, Osborn RS. Crystalline composition of equine urinary calculi. Res Vet Sci 1986; 40(3):288–91.
[17] Hope WD, Wilsom JH, Hager DA, et al. Chronic renal failure associated with bilateral nephroliths and ureteroliths in a two-year-old Thoroughbred colt. Equine Vet J 1989;21(3): 228–31.
[18] Kaneps AJ, Shires GMH, Watrous BJ. Cystic calculi in two horses. J Am Vet Med Assoc 1985;187(7):737–9.
[19] Brück I, Hesselholt M. Nephrolithiasis als Kolikursache beim Pferd. Tierarztl Prax 1992; 20(6):611–4 [in German].
[20] van Dongen PL, Plenderleith RW. Equine urolithiasis: surgical treatment by Gökel's pararectal cystotomy. Equine Veterinary Education 1994;6(4):186–8.

[21] Röcken M, Stehle C, Mosel G, et al. Laparoscopic-assisted cystotomy for urolith removal in geldings. Vet Surg 2006;35(4):394–7.

[22] Diaz-Espineira M, Escolar E, Bellanato J, et al. Infrared and anatomic spectrometry analysis of the mineral composition of a series of equine sabulous material samples and urinary calculi. Res Vet Sci 1997;63(2):93–5.

[23] Mair TS, McCaig J. Cystic calculus in a horse. Equine Vet J 1983;15(2):173–4.

[24] Moore S, Gowland G. The immunologic integrity of matrix substance A and its possible detection and quantitation in urine. Br J Urol 1975;47(5):489–94.

[25] Wickham JEA. The matrix of renal calculi. In: Williams DI, Chishold GO, editors. Scientific foundations of urology, vol. 1. Chicago: Year Book Medical Publishers; 1976. p. 323–9.

[26] Rose AG, Sulaman S. Tamm-Horsfall mucoproteins promote calcium oxalate crystal formation in urine: quantitative studies. J Urol 1982;127(1):177–9.

[27] Mair TS, Osborn RS. Crystalline composition of normal equine urine deposits. Equine Vet J 1990;22(5):364–5.

[28] Wood T, Weckman TJ, Henry PA, et al. Equine urine pH: normal population distributions and methods of acidification. Equine Vet J 1990;22(2):118–21.

[29] De Yoreo JJ, Qiu SR, Hoyer JR. Molecular modulation of calcium oxalate crystallization. Am J Physiol Renal Physiol 2006;291(6):F1123–32.

[30] Senior DF, Finlayson B. Initiation and growth of uroliths. Vet Clin North Am Small Anim Pract 1986;16(1):19–26.

[31] Schumacher J, Schumacher J. Surgical management of urolithiasis in the equine male. In: Wolfe DF, Moll HD, editors. Large animal urogenital surgery. 2nd edition. Baltimore (MD): Williams & Wilkins; 1999. p. 69–73.

[32] Textor JA, Slone DE, Clark CK. Cystolithiasis secondary to intravesical foreign body in a horse. Vet Rec 2005;156(1):24–6.

[33] Rodger LD, Carlson GP, Moran ME, et al. Resolution of a left ureteral stone using electrohydraulic lithotripsy in a thoroughbred colt. J Vet Intern Med 1995;9(4):280–2.

[34] Ryall LR. Macromolecules and urolithiasis: parallels and paradoxes. Nephron Physiol 2004; 98(2):37–42.

[35] Carvalho M, Lulich JP, Osborne CA, et al. Defective urinary crystallization inhibition and urinary stone formation. Int Braz J Urol 2006;32(3):342–9.

[36] Gill WB, Jones KW, Ruggiero KJ. Protective effects of heparin and other sulfated glycosaminoglycans on crystal adhesion to injured urothelium. J Urol 1982;127(1):152–4.

[37] Khan SR, Cockrell CA, Finlayson B, et al. Crystal retention by injured urothelium on the rat urinary bladder. J Urol 1984;132(1):153–7.

[38] Parsons CL, Stauffer C, Schmidt JD. Bladder-surface glycosaminoglycans: an efficient mechanism of environmental adaptation. Science 1980;208(4444):605–7.

[39] Hanson RR, Poland HM. Perineal urethrotomy for removal of cystic calculi in a gelding. J Am Vet Med Assoc 1995;207(4):418–9.

[40] Beard W. Parainguinal laparocystotomy for urolith removal in geldings. Vet Surg 2004; 33(4):386–90.

[41] Wooldridge AA, Seahorn TL, Williams J, et al. Chronic renal failure associated with nephrolithiasis, ureterolithiasis, and renal dysplasia in a 2-year-old quarter horse gelding. Vet Radiol Ultrasound 1999;40(4):361–4.

[42] Byars TD, Simpson JS, Divers TJ, et al. Percutaneous nephrostomy in short-term management of ureterolithiasis and renal dysfunction in a filly. J Am Vet Med Assoc 1989;195(4): 499–501.

[43] Newton SA, Cheeseman MT, Edwards GB. Bilateral renal and ureteral calculi in a 10-year-old gelding. Vet Rec 1999;144(13):383–5.

[44] DeBowes RM. Surgical management of urolithiasis. Vet Clin North Am Equine Pract 1988; 4(3):461–71.

[45] Rantanen NW. Diseases of the kidneys. Vet Clin North Am Large Anim Pract 1986;16(2): 89–103.

[46] Trotter GW, Brown CM, Ainsworth DM. Unilateral nephrectomy for treatment of a renal abscess in a foal. J Am Vet Med Assoc 1984;184(11):1392–4.
[47] Jones SL, Langer LL, Sterner-Kock A, et al. Renal dysplasia and benign ureteropelvic polyps associated with hydronephrosis in a foal. J Am Vet Med Assoc 1994;204(8): 1230–4.
[48] Keoughan CG, Rodgerson DH, Brown MP. Hand-assisted laparoscopic left nephrectomy in standing horses. Vet Surg 2003;206(3):206–12.
[49] Lillich JD, Fischer AT Jr, DeBowes RM. Kidneys and ureters. In: Auer JA, Stick JA, editors. Equine surgery. 3rd edition. St. Louis (MO): Saunders/Elsevier; 2006. p. 870–7.
[50] Mitchell KJ, Dowling BA, Hughes KJ, et al. Unilateral nephrectomy as a treatment for renal trauma in a foal. Aust Vet J 2004;82(12):753–5.
[51] Marien T. Laparoscopic nephrectomy in the standing horse. In: Fischer AT Jr, editor. Equine diagnostic and surgical laparoscopy. Philadelphia: WB Saunders; 2002. p. 273–81.
[52] Lillich JD, Fischer AT Jr, DeBowes RM. Bladder. In: Auer JA, Stick JA, editors. Equine surgery. 3rd edition. St. Louis (MO): Saunders/Elsevier; 2006. p. 877–87.
[53] Ragle CA. Dorsally recumbent urinary endoscopic surgery. Vet Clin North Am Equine Pract 2000;16(2):343–50.
[54] Hackett R. Vesical calculi. In: Mansmann R, McAllister E, editors. Equine medicine and surgery. Santa Barbara (CA): American Veterinary Publications; 1982. p. 913–8.
[55] Howard RD, Pleasant RS, May KA. Pulsed dye laser lithotripsy for treatment of urolithiasis in two geldings. J Am Vet Med Assoc 1998;212(10):1600–3.
[56] May KA, Pleasant RS, Howard RD, et al. Failure of holmium:yttrium-aluminum-garnet laser lithotripsy in two horses with calculi in the urinary bladder. J Am Vet Med Assoc 2001;219(7):957–61.
[57] Judy CE, Galuppo LD. Endoscopic-assisted disruption of urinary calculi using a holmium: YAG laser in standing horses. Vet Surg 2002;31(3):245–50.
[58] Simhofer H, Riedelberger K. Endoscopic lithotripsy of a large cystic calculus with a holmium-YAG-laser in a gelding. Dtsch Tierarztl Wochenschr 2002;109(9):383–6.
[59] Hanson K. Minimally invasive and surgical management of urinary stones. Urol Nurs 2005; 25(6):458–64.
[60] Gayer G, Hertz M, Stav K, et al. Minimally invasive management of urolithiasis. Semin Ultrasound CT MR 2006;27(6):139–51.
[61] Adams LG, Senior DF. Electrohydraulic and extracorporeal shock-wave lithotripsy. Vet Clin North Am Small Anim Pract 1999;29(1):293–302.
[62] MacHarg MA, Foerner JJ, Phillips TN, et al. Electrohydraulic lithotripsy for treatment of a cystic calculus in a mare. Vet Surg 1985;14(4):325–7.
[63] Eustace RA, Hunt JM, Brearley MJ. Electrohydraulic lithotripsy for the treatment of cystic calculus in two geldings. Equine Vet J 1988;20(3):221–3.
[64] Koenig J, Hurtig M, Pearce S, et al. Ballistic shock wave lithotripsy in an 18-year-old Thoroughbred gelding. Can Vet J 1999;40(3):185–6.
[65] Keeley FX Jr, Pillai M, Smith M, et al. Electrokinetic lithotripsy: safety, efficacy and limitations of a new form of ballistic lithotripsy. BJU Int 1999;84(3):261–3.
[66] Menezes P, Kumar PVS, Timoney AG. A randomized trial comparing lithoclast with an electrokinetic lithotripter in the management of ureteric stones. BJU Int 2000;85(1):22–5.
[67] Remillard RL, Modransky PD, Welker FH, et al. Dietary management of cystic calculi in a horse. J Equine Vet Sci 1992;12(6):359–63.
[68] Firth EC. Urethral sphincterotomy for delivery of a vesical calculus in the mare: a case report. Equine Vet J 1976;8(3):99–100.
[69] Nicoletta JA, Lande MB. Medical evaluation and treatment of urolithiasis. Pediatr Clin North Am 2006;53(3):479–91.
[70] Dusterdieck KF, Schott HC 2nd, Eberhart SW, et al. Electrolyte and glycerol supplementation improve water intake by horses performing a simulated 60 km endurance ride. Equine Vet J Suppl 1999;30:418–24.

[71] Diaz-Espineira M, Escolar E, Bellanato J, et al. Crystalline composition of equine urinary sabulous deposits. Scanning Microsc 1995;9(4):1071–9.
[72] Diaz-Espineira M, Escolar E, Bellanato J, et al. Minor constituents of sabulous material in equine urine. Res Vet Sci 1996;60(3):238–42.
[73] Adams LG, Dollahite JW, Romane WM, et al. Cystitis and ataxia associated with sorghum ingestion by horses. J Am Vet Med Assoc 1969;155(3):518–24.

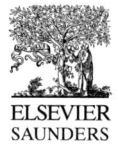

VETERINARY
CLINICS
Equine Practice

Vet Clin Equine 23 (2007) 631–639

Equine Renal Tubular Disorders

Luis G. Arroyo, DVM, DVSc[a],
Henry R. Stämpfli, DVM, DrMedVet[b],*

[a]Department of Pathobiology, Ontario Veterinary College, University of Guelph,
Guelph, Ontario, Canada, N1G 2W1
[b]Department of Clinical Studies, Ontario Veterinary College, University of Guelph,
Guelph, Ontario, Canada, N1G 2W1

Renal tubular disorders have been sporadically reported in horses. Only three types of tubular defects have been recognized: (1) nephrogenic diabetes insipidus, attributed to unresponsiveness of the renal tubules to antidiuretic hormone; (2) distal renal tubular acidosis (RTA; type I); and (3) proximal RTA (type II) [1–4]. The following review focuses on RTA and nephrogenic diabetes insipidus.

Renal tubular acidoses

RTAs are forms of metabolic acidoses thought to arise from a lack of urine excretion of protons or loss of bicarbonate ions because of a variety of tubular disorders. They are clinically characterized by a metabolic hyperchloremic (non-anion gap) acidosis without impaired glomerular filtration. Molecular studies have identified genetic or acquired defects in proton and bicarbonate transporters with additional involvement of chloride and sodium transporters. A few cases have been associated with primary defects primarily in electrolyte transporters. There are multiple forms of RTA identified and described in people (types I, II, and IV), but only type I and II have been reported but poorly differentiated in horses. There is no breed or gender predisposition in horses, nor is there any evidence that environment or diet could predispose to the development of this condition. Central to RTA are the kidneys and their role in acid-base regulation. It seems appropriate to review the physiology briefly by comparing traditional and quantitative acid-base interpretation theories.

* Corresponding author.
E-mail address: hstaempf@uoguelph.ca (H.R. Stämpfli).

Kidney as regulator of acid-base balance

Classic acid-base interpretation

The traditional model of acid-base balance and its interpretation assumes that the balance between hydrogen ion generation and urinary secretion determines plasma H^+ concentration. The renal contribution in maintaining the acid-base homeostasis occurs as a result of the reabsorption of filtered bicarbonate (HCO_3^-) HCO_3^-, mainly at the level of the proximal convoluted tubule (Fig. 1), and through the excretion of titrated acids in urinary buffers and the excretion of ammonium (NH_4^+) at the level of the distal nephron (Fig. 2) [5]. Proximal bicarbonate reabsorption is, however, incompletely understood [6]. The daily acid production is calculated as the combined excretion of inorganic (SO_4^{2-}) and organic anions in the urine. Renal elimination of acid equivalents is computed as the combined titrable acidity plus NH_4^+ minus the excreted HCO_3^-, which is called net acid excretion (NAE). Central to the renal acid-base physiology, when using the classic acid-base interpretation, is the excretion of NH_4^+ through a complicated network of transport mechanisms outside the scope of this article (NH_4^+ transporters, influence of NH_4^+ on other tubular processes involved in

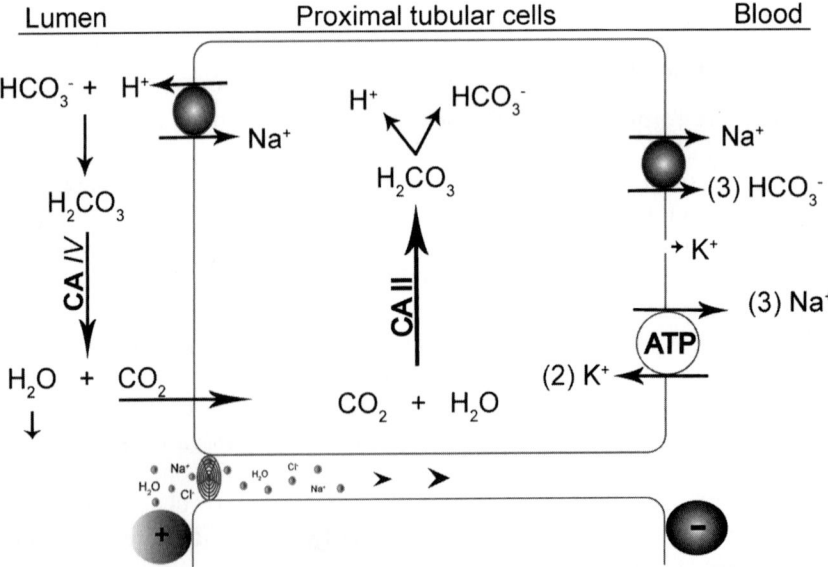

Fig. 1. Traditional model of the transport mechanisms involved in bicarbonate reabsorption in the proximal tubule. H^+ secretion occurs at the apical membrane by means of an Na^+/H^+ exchanger and HCO_3^- is transported at the basolateral membrane by means of an Na/ HCO_3^- cotransporter. The bicarbonate absorption process is catalyzed in the proximal tubule by the carbonic anhydrase II (CA II) and carbonic anhydrase IV (CA IV) in the cytoplasm and luminal space, respectively.

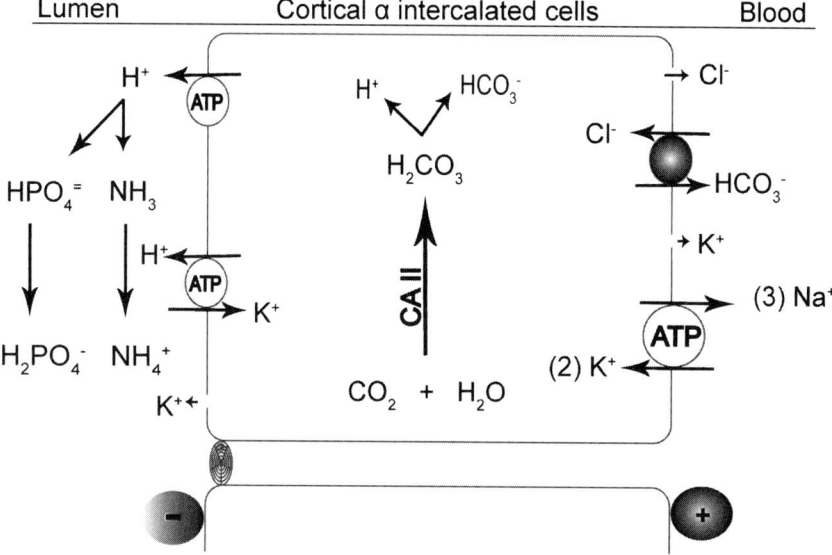

Fig. 2. Schematic illustration of the traditional model for H^+ secretion in the distal collecting tubules. H^+ is actively secreted into the tubular lumen by means of an ATPase pump, and bicarbonate leaves the cells at the basolateral border by means of a Cl^-/HCO_3^- exchanger. Cytoplasmic carbonic anhydrase II (CA II) catalyzed the formation of proton and bicarbonate.

acid-base regulation). Why NH_4^+ excretion is important to acid-base homeostasis in the kidneys is not entirely clear, however.

Physicochemical (quantitative) acid-base interpretation

The traditional acid-base interpretation has been complemented more recently by a quantitative approach to acid-base balance interpretation called the physicochemical approach to acid base (Stewart method). This approach is based on laws of conservation of mass, dissociation equilibria, and electroneutrality in biologic watery solutions. It uses the concept of completely dissociated strong ions (Na^+, K^+, Cl^-, Ca^{++}, Mg^{++}, SO_4^-, and lactate), partially dissociated weak acids (mainly proteins and phosphate [blood] and, additionally, NH_4^+ in urine), and volatile buffers (carbonate species) [7]. Three independent variables are taken into account: the strong ions as strong ion difference (SID) (SID $= Na^+ + K^+ - Cl^-$), the total concentration of weak acids (A_{tot}; mostly plasma proteins, including phosphate buffer system), and P_{CO_2}. The kidney plays a central role in acid-base homeostasis by adjusting urine electrolyte excretion to maintain constant osmolarity and electrolyte body balance. Strictly applying physicochemical principles, to look at the physiology of renal handling of acids and bases, it boils down to renal regulation of the independent variable strong electrolytes (sodium [Na], potassium [K], and chlorine [Cl]), p_{CO_2}, and, to a lesser degree, weak acids—nothing more and nothing less. Examples are the use of ammonium chloride in animals to manipulate urinary pH or the dietary cation anion balance (DCAB) in cattle to change endogenous acid production to assist in control of periparturient hypocalcemia. Ingestion of a low-DCAB diet induces a strong ion (metabolic) acidosis [8], as indicated by a decreased plasma SID and bicarbonate concentration, a decreased urinary pH, and an increased NAE [9,10]. The use of the quantitative acid-base approach also looks closely at the cationic side of the acid-base balance and postulates different pathophysiologic mechanisms for acid-base derangements compared with traditional pH and anionic-centered approaches.

Pathogenesis

Proximal renal tubular acidosis (type II)

In this form of the disorder, the classic explanation proposes that dysfunctional proximal tubular cells are unable to reabsorb bicarbonate, resulting in a net loss of bicarbonate in the urine. Normally, hydrogen ions are secreted and bicarbonate is reabsorbed, but when this function is impaired, metabolic acidosis ensues. The serum bicarbonate decreases to a level of equilibrium at which the tubule is able to reclaim the reduced filtered bicarbonate but the serum bicarbonate level remains low [11]. The acidification mechanisms in the distal tubules are not affected; therefore, the daily acid load is successfully excreted. Defective reabsorption of glucose, amino acids, electrolytes, and organic acids can also occur; in such cases, the condition is better known as Fanconi syndrome. In people, proximal RTA can be inherited or acquired. This syndrome can be inherited as an autosomal dominant or autosomal recessive trait or as a gender-linked disorder (X chromosome). Most of the inherited cases of isolated proximal RTA are autosomal dominant. These patients can never reach a normal serum pH, but they seem to respond well when treated with oral sodium bicarbonate and have normal proximal tubular function test results. The molecular basis of the genetic defect in these patients has not been determined. Acquired isolated proximal RTA may occur as a result of medications that inhibit carbonic anhydrase (eg, acetazolamide).

Applying the physiochemical approach to explain hyperchloremic acidosis in type II RTA, the condition is caused by retention of chloride ions changing the equation for electroneutrality and passively decreasing bicarbonate concentrations in serum (concept of independent versus dependent variables). The major difference between the two schools of thoughts regarding the acid-base balance is that the classic approach is pH centered and the quantitative approach is electrolyte centered. Future research is needed to elucidate the pathophysiology of proximal RTA using the quantitative approach. In addition to the classic proton pump research, efforts should concentrate on investigating channel dysfunctions of strong electrolytes [12].

Distal renal tubular acidosis (type I)

Using the classic approach, the distal nephron is not capable of lowering the urine pH normally because there is an excessive back diffusion of H^+ ion from the lumen to the blood stream or because of inadequate transport of H^+ at the level of the collecting ducts. The impaired secretion of NH_4^+ is secondary to this defect. The reabsorption of bicarbonate is quantitatively normal; however, as a result of the elevated urine pH, some degree of bicarbonaturia is present.

Human patients with nephrocalcinosis or urolithiasis have a condition often called incomplete distal RTA. Those patients are unable to acidify urine, but a high rate of NH_4^+ excretion compensates for the limited excretion of acid. Distal RTA is the more common form of inherited RTA. Dominant and recessive forms exist, and the latter may occur with or without deafness. Recent research has concentrated on anion exchangers (chloride/bicarbonate) defects. A rare drug-related form of distal RTA with hypokalemia may be induced with amphotericin B treatment, and sometimes with cyclosporine A treatment, in human patients.

The physicochemical interpretation of distal RTA again concentrates mostly on strong electrolyte, especially chloride handling, disorders in the distal tubule. It could well be that urine pH is not decreasing with increased chloride excretion, because potassium might also be excreted at an increased level. It is now known that urinary pH is mainly determined by SID.

Risk factors

In people, some cases can be congenital, acquired, or idiopathic. Several drugs have been attributed to induced RTA type II and are also widely used in horses; among these drugs are aminoglycosides, tetracyclines, trimethoprim/sulfamethoxazole, carbonic anhydrase inhibitors, amphotericin B, nonsteroidal anti-inflammatory drugs, and lithium carbonate. Other possible causes suggested in horses included pyelonephritis, hyperparathyroidism, and hypervitaminosis D.

Clinical signs

Common reported clinical signs in horses include depression, poor performance, weight loss, anorexia, weakness, colic, decreased gastrointestinal motility, decreased fecal output, dehydration, poor condition, tachycardia, tachypnea, and ataxia in addition to polyuria and polydipsia. People who have hypokalemic distal RTA frequently complain of musculoskeletal conditions, such as arthralgia, myalgia, muscle weakness, or low back pain.

Diagnosis

Adequate approaches to suspected cases of RTA include a detailed clinical history; physical examination; and venous blood gas analysis, including electrolytes and a biochemistry profile. Additional tests are imperative to differentiate the type of RTA. In general, RTA should be considered in horses presented with hyperchloremic metabolic acidosis with a normal plasma anion gap, especially in those cases with no evidence of sodium bicarbonate losses (ie, gastrointestinal) or exogenous acid administration (parenteral saline overload).

Blood gas and electrolyte analyses show hyperchloremia, metabolic acidosis, and low SID. Serum chloride levels can range from 106 to 121 mEq/L, and bicarbonate concentrations are often less than 13 mEq/L. Other electrolyte abnormalities, such as hyponatremia and hypokalemia, have been reported in some equine cases. Azotemia from prerenal and renal damage has been confirmed in several cases; however, the initiating cause of renal damage is usually undetermined.

In human patients, precise recognition of the type of RTA is important in terms of treatment, severity, and prognosis. Distal RTA is characterized by the inability to decrease urine pH to less than 5.5 despite metabolic acidosis and the inability to augment NH_4^+ excretion. Proximal RTA is characterized by a bicarbonate wasting state because of impaired reabsorption in the proximal tubule, but the ability to acidify the urine in the distal tubule remains intact. Therefore, when the plasma HCO_3^- declines, also decreasing the amount of HCO_3^- filtered, the urine pH becomes acid. Differentiation between RTA I and II is difficult, unreliable, and clinically not important in horses. In addition, urine pH in horses is normally alkaline (pH 7–9), and some ancillary tests that can be used are mentioned briefly here.

HCO_3^- titration

This test measures the rate of reabsorption and excretion of bicarbonate at different filtered loads. Sodium bicarbonate is infused intravenously to produce small increments in plasma concentration; simultaneously, the concentrations of bicarbonate and creatinine are measured in blood and urine. The rates of reabsorption and excretion are compared with the corresponding values of plasma. The calculation of the renal bicarbonate threshold gives the necessary information for the diagnosis of a tubular defect to reabsorb bicarbonate. This test has not been described in horses.

Ammonium chloride challenge

The ability of the distal tube to excrete hydrogen ions under normal physiologic circumstances can be used to distinguish RTA I and II. Ammonium chloride, 0.1 g/kg of body weight, diluted in 6 L of water is administered per nasogastric intubation. Normally, urine acidification should occur;

therefore, the inability to lower the urine pH (<6.5) would be consistent with distal RTA. Also, when the concentrations of P_{CO_2}, total carbon dioxide (T_{CO_2}), and HCO_3^- in urine are higher compared with blood, a reabsorption defect is suspected and is consistent with proximal RTA.

When applying physicochemical interpretation to these RTA diagnostic tests, the sodium and chloride handling of the renal tubules becomes central, including a different pathophysiologic interpretation.

Treatment

The objective of treatment is directed to correct the biochemical abnormalities and to improve general health and prevent the progression or development of other complications.

In human patients, oral alkali tablets are used most commonly (sodium-bicarbonate or sodium/potassium-citrate). The amount of the sodium alkali administered should compensate for the urinary loss of sodium bicarbonate and the amount of acid generated as a result of protein catabolism and growth (young animals). Currently, horses with RTA are treated with intravenous and oral administration of sodium bicarbonate, and the deficit can usually be corrected within 24 hours. The sodium bicarbonate deficit is calculated using the following formula:

$$\text{Total Body NaHCO}_3^- \text{ Deficit (mEq)}$$
$$\text{(as reported on the blood gas report)}$$
$$\times \text{ Body Weight (kg)} \times \text{ Volume of Distribution}$$
$$\times \text{ Serum HCO}_3^- \text{ Deficit}$$

One caveat is that the base deficit reported on blood gas results is usually corrected by the machine used to human normal values of blood bicarbonate concentrations of 24 mEq/L and not to normal levels of horses, which are usually 28 to 32 mEq/L for venous blood samples.

Commonly, horses with RTA are dehydrated and azotemic; therefore, adequate fluid therapy to correct and maintain normal hydration and to establish diuresis is part of the immediate therapy plan. Hypokalemia may be present in RTA cases or may develop during correction of the metabolic acidosis. Potassium can be added to the initial fluid therapy (20–40 mEq/L), not to exceed an administration rate of 0.5 mEq/kg/h, and is supplemented orally after initial intravenous treatment, preferably in the form of potassium citrate or bicarbonate rather than chloride.

Prognosis

There are reports of spontaneous recovery in horses with distal RTA. Recurrence has been reported to occur within days to years after diagnosis, and successful treatment has been reported in a high proportion of horses (63%). Recurrence was found to occur more commonly in animals with underlying renal disease, however. Therefore, the short-term prognosis may seem favorable, but future complications can usually be expected in cases with underlying renal disease. The long-term effect of sodium bicarbonate supplementation in horses is currently unknown. The authors currently have a Fresian horse (female, 3.5 years of age) diagnosed with RTA, which has been on oral sodium-bicarbonate supplementation for more than 2 years, without adverse side effects. This horse has shown normal growth and weight gain rates compared with herd mates.

Nephrogenic diabetes insipidus

This rare disorder of horses consists of the inability to concentrate the urine as a result of failure by the collection ducts to respond to vasopressin. This condition may be acquired or inherited, and the congenital form is linked to male gender in people. The acquired form is seen in horses with damaged renal tubules caused by aminoglycosides, nonsteroidal anti-inflammatory drugs, and particularly tetracyclines. Additional causes include pyelonephritis, oxalate toxicity, and blister beetle toxicity.

Nephrogenic diabetes insipidus has been diagnosed in three colts, of which two were full thoroughbred siblings. The most remarkable clinical signs are a history of excessive urination and extreme polydipsia (PU/PD). Other findings include thin body condition, rough hair coat, and small stature (growth retardation).

The diagnosis of nephrogenic diabetes insipidus has been based on the inability to concentrate urine in response to water deprivation, infusion of hypertonic saline, or exogenous vasopressin administration, which is indicative of insensitivity of the collecting duct epithelial cells to vasopressin. Plasma vasopressin concentration after water deprivation is expected to increase.

Treatment is directed at managing the PU/PD. The treatment of choice in human patients is restricted sodium and water intake and administration of thiazide diuretics [3,13].

References

[1] Trotter GW, Miller D, Parks A, et al. Type II renal tubular acidosis in a mare. J Am Vet Med Assoc 1986;188(9):1050–1.
[2] Aleman MR, Kuesis B, Schott HC, et al. Renal tubular acidosis in horses (1980–1999). J Vet Intern Med 2001;15(2):136–43.
[3] Schott HC 2nd, Bayly WM, Reed SM, et al. Nephrogenic diabetes insipidus in sibling colts. J Vet Intern Med 1993;7(2):68–72.
[4] Gull T. Type 1 renal tubular acidosis in a broodmare. Vet Clin North Am Equine Pract 2006; 22(1):229–37.
[5] Rodriguez Soriano J. Renal tubular acidosis: the clinical entity. J Am Soc Nephrol 2002; 13(8):2160–70.

[6] Weinstein AM. Mathematical models of renal fluid and electrolyte transport: acknowledging our uncertainty. Am J Physiol Renal Physiol 2003;284(5):F871–84.

[7] Corey HE, Vallo A, Rodriguez-Soriano J. An analysis of renal tubular acidosis by the Stewart method. Pediatr Nephrol 2006;21(2):206–11.

[8] Constable PD. Clinical assessment of acid-base status. Strong ion difference theory. Vet Clin North Am Food Anim Pract 1999;15(3):447–71.

[9] Tucker WB, Harrison GA, Hemken RW, et al. Efficacy of simulated, slow release sodium bicarbonate in stabilizing ruminal milieu and acid-base status in lactating dairy cattle. J Dairy Sci 1988;71(7):1823–9.

[10] Vagnoni DB, Oetzel GR. Effects of dietary cation-anion difference on the acid-base status of dry cows. J Dairy Sci 1998;81(6):1643–52.

[11] Rocher LL, Tannen RL. The clinical spectrum of renal tubular acidosis. Annu Rev Med 1986;37:319–31.

[12] Ring T, Frische S, Nielsen S. Clinical review: renal tubular acidosis—a physicochemical approach. Crit Care 2005;9(6):573–80.

[13] Brashier M. Polydipsia and polyuria in a weanling colt caused by nephrogenic diabetes insipidus. Vet Clin North Am Equine Pract 2006;22(1):219–27.

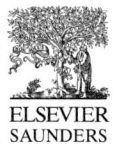

ELSEVIER
SAUNDERS

VETERINARY
CLINICS
Equine Practice

Vet Clin Equine 23 (2007) 641–653

Polyuria and Polydipsia in Horses

Erica C. McKenzie, BSc, BVMS, PhD

*Clinical Sciences Department, College of Veterinary Medicine, Oregon State University,
227 Magruder Hall, Corvallis, OR 97331, USA*

Polyuria and polydipsia, although infrequently reported in horses, can create considerable inconvenience for the owners of stabled horses and pose a unique diagnostic challenge for the clinician. Although the two conditions usually occur simultaneously, because water intake and excretion are closely linked, it is important for the clinician to distinguish the primary issue correctly to determine appropriate therapy and management and to provide an accurate prognosis for resolution or recovery.

Water balance in the healthy horse

Water intake and urine production

Healthy horses require between 25 and 70 mL/kg of body weight in water per day to meet maintenance water requirements [1–3]. Requirements are met largely by means of the water content of food and, to a smaller extent, by means of the production of metabolic water from the catabolism of fats, protein, and carbohydrate, with remaining requirements met through drinking [4,5]. The amount of water consumed per day is heavily influenced by dietary composition and physiologic demands, including lactation and exercise, which may increase water requirements 50% to 400% depending on various factors, including exercise intensity, ambient temperature, and humidity [4,6].

Water intake in sedentary horses correlates strongly to dry matter intake and is largely a periprandial phenomenon, with most drinking activity reported to occur within 10 minutes before and 30 minutes after eating [7]. Horses usually consume 3 to 4 L of water per kilogram of hay dry matter, although lower rates of water intake may be observed in donkeys and ponies [8,9]. Water requirements increase as the digestibility of feed sources

---

E-mail address: erica.mckenzie@oregonstate.edu

decreases to compensate for increased fecal water losses resulting from greater fecal mass. Hence, water requirements are higher for horses consuming hay versus grain-based rations [2,4]. Horses subsisting on growing forage may meet water requirements entirely through feed intake because of the high moisture content of pasture [4]. Additional voluntary water consumption is likely if water is available, however. Failure to meet water requirements results in decreased dry matter intake and potentially decreased performance [4,10].

Healthy horses usually produce urine at a rate of 15 to 30 mL/kg/d, resulting in a daily urine volume of approximately 5 to 15 L [1,3,5,11–13]. A considerably wider range of daily urine volume (2–26 L) has been reported in healthy horses, however, influenced by dietary composition and feed and water intake [14,15]. Foals have a relatively greater urine output for their body size than mature horses, with reported urine volumes of 2.6 to 8.6 L/d (148 mL/kg of body weight per day) [16]. This is likely attributable to the fact that hyposthenuria develops rapidly within 12 hours of birth in foals and persists for the first 6 to 8 weeks of life, associated with consumption of a milk diet and a lower renal solute load [17,18].

Maintenance of water balance

Water homeostasis largely depends on the actions of antidiuretic hormone (ADH) and, to a lesser degree, on the renin-angiotensin-aldosterone system [19]. ADH produced within the supraoptic and paraventricular nuclei of the hypothalamus is stored within the posterior pituitary and released primarily in response to increased plasma osmolality sensed by hypothalamic osmoreceptors [20]. ADH acts on the distal renal tubule and collecting ducts to promote the absorption of water into the renal medullary interstitium, with the subsequent production of more concentrated urine [19–21]. Angiotensin II is produced as the end result of renin release from the renal juxtaglomerular cells in response to decreased circulating volume. Angiotensin II directly stimulates sodium and water resorption in the proximal renal tubule in addition to prompting aldosterone release, which subsequently stimulates sodium resorption in the distal renal tubule. Angiotensin II is also partially responsible for stimulation of thirst [19].

Successful conservation of water therefore depends on successful production and release of ADH in response to appropriate stimuli, sensitivity of the nephrons to the actions of ADH, a minimum number of functioning nephrons (at least one third of the nephrons must be functional), and the presence of a hypertonic renal medullary interstitium [21,22]. Disruption at any level may impede the ability to respond to changes in water balance and can subsequently result in polyuria and polydipsia.

In a mature horse with a body weight of 500 kg, polydipsia (excessive water intake) is suggested to correspond to the consumption of 50 L (100 mL/kg/d) or more of water per day and polyuria (excessive urine volume) to the production of 25 L (50 mL/kg/d) or more of urine, figures that are partly based on extrapolation from cats and dogs [23]. When attempting to establish if polyuria or polydipsia is truly occurring, however, all factors capable of influencing water intake and excretion must be considered. Water intake can be profound but appropriate with certain physiologic demands, and urine volumes of this magnitude are occasionally reported in apparently healthy horses [15]. Horses exercising in a warm environment or encountering substantial water losses because of colonic disease may consume water in excess of 100 L/d without a corresponding increase in urine volume [24]. Accurate demonstration of polyuria and polydipsia must therefore rely on objective and, whenever possible, repeated measurements of water consumption or urine production, with thorough assessment of any factors that may potentially influence these two variables.

Causes of polydipsia and polyuria

Polydipsia

Primary polydipsia in species other than the horse has been attributed to psychogenic disorders and to disorders of the hypothalamic thirst center [19,20,22]. In horses, primary polydipsia is believed to reflect a psychogenic tendency to consume excessive amounts of water, resulting in secondary polyuria [9,25]. Psychogenic polydipsia is probably the most common cause of excessive water intake and excessive urination in mature stabled horses, likely as a result of confinement and boredom [26]. The degree of polydipsia and polyuria in afflicted horses is often extreme. Hyposthenuria is present (urine specific gravity <1.005), but no other physical abnormalities are usually noted [23,27].

Excessive voluntary salt consumption (psychogenic salt consumption) has also been proposed as a cause of polydipsia in the horse but reflects a compensatory response to polyuria induced by solute diuresis [28–30]. Equine rations typically contain a negligible amount of salt in the absence of extravagant dietary supplementation [31]. Occasionally, however, an individual horse may display voluntary consumption of unusually large amounts of salt, associated with polydipsia [29]. It is likely that salt consumption would have to exceed 5% of dry matter intake to induce a polydipsic effect, and concurrent clinical signs, including muscle tremors and a stiff gait, may be observed [23,29,32].

Polyuria

Pathologic polyuria can arise from primary renal disturbances or from systemic disease syndromes. Primary renal disturbances causing polyuria in the horse include renal failure and nephrogenic diabetes insipidus [33,34]. Iatrogenic polyuria is associated with the administration of intravenous fluids, corticosteroids, diuretics, and other pharmacologic agents with a direct action on the kidney, including α_2-adrenoceptor agonist drugs [23,26,35]. The most frequent systemic disease syndrome associated with polyuria in horses is pituitary pars intermedia dysfunction (PPID or equine Cushing's disease), although polyuria does not seem to be a consistent finding in all cases [23,26,36,37]. Additionally, neurogenic (central) diabetes insipidus, diabetes mellitus, and endotoxemia may be associated with polyuria in horses [23,26].

Chronic renal failure is one of the more common causes of polyuria in horses [27]. A decrease in the number of functional renal tubules promotes increased loss of urinary solute accompanied by an obligatory increase in water loss as increasing amounts of glomerular filtrate are presented to remaining nephron segments, exceeding their absorptive capacity. Decreased renal medullary hypertonicity and an impaired response of renal collecting ducts to ADH may represent additional contributing factors [19,38]. Although the initiating cause of renal dysfunction is often not able to be determined at the time that clinical signs of chronic renal failure are recognized, potential causes include glomerulonephritis, congenital renal abnormalities, amyloidosis, pyelonephritis, urinary obstruction, neoplasia and progression of acute renal failure initiated by hemodynamic disturbances, nephrotoxin exposure, severe endotoxemia, pigmenturia, and others [33,39].

Nephrogenic diabetes insipidus is characterized by failure of the renal tubules to respond to ADH, effectively preventing renal conservation of water in response to water deprivation or exogenous ADH administration [20]. Primary nephrogenic diabetes insipidus is a rare cause of polyuria in the horse but has been described as an apparently familial trait in two related Thoroughbred horses with profound polydipsia [34]. Affected horses became dehydrated during water restriction and maintained hyposthenuric or isosthenuric urine specific gravity after administration of exogenous ADH. Plasma ADH concentrations became elevated in response to water restriction in the one horse in which they were measured, confirming a diagnosis of nephrogenic rather than central diabetes insipidus [34]. Decreased renal responsiveness to ADH most commonly represents a secondary event related to underlying disease, however, including renal failure and a variety of endocrine and metabolic disorders [20,22].

Central or neurogenic diabetes insipidus reflects a failure of production or release of ADH, resulting in profound polydipsia/polyuria and the production of hyposthenuric urine [5,19]. In human beings and small animal species, neurogenic diabetes insipidus is occasionally congenital and frequently idiopathic in nature, and it has also been reported in association with trauma, intracranial neoplasia, and inflammatory diseases [20,40,41]. Complete neurogenic diabetes insipidus has been described in two horses as an idiopathic syndrome or in association with encephalitis [42,43]. The affected horses were unable to concentrate urine appropriately in response to water deprivation but responded to exogenously administered ADH.

A lack of increase in plasma ADH concentration in response to water deprivation was documented in one horse in which plasma ADH was measured, further supporting the diagnosis of central diabetes insipidus [42]. Polyuria and polydipsia are often reported in horses with PPID, possibly as a result of impingement of the abnormal pars intermedia tissue on the hypothalamus and pituitary interfering with ADH production or release, resulting in a syndrome of partial neurogenic diabetes insipidus [28,36,37]. Pituitary neoplasia is reported in a significant proportion of dogs with central diabetes insipidus [41]. Other factors that may contribute to the occurrence of polyuria in horses with PPID include osmotic diuresis associated with glucosuria and antagonism of ADH action at the renal tubule associated with increased plasma cortisol concentration [23,26].

Although the occurrence of glucosuria, hyperglycemia, and polydipsia/polyuria in horses is usually indicative of PPID, diabetes mellitus unrelated to PPID is occasionally described as a cause of these findings [44–48]. Polyuria and polydipsia in diabetes mellitus are attributable to glucosuria and can be profound [19,46].

In small animal species, polyuria/polydipsia is reported in association with liver disease, potentially as a result of increased endogenous corticosteroid concentrations, a primary polydipsic effect, or reduced renal medullary tonicity attributable to impaired urea formation [19,21]. Steroid hepatopathy has been reported as a cause of polydipsia and polyuria in horses, but the polyuria possibly reflects the effects of the exogenously administered corticosteroids rather than liver dysfunction per se [49,50].

Septic conditions, most notably pyometra of the bitch, are associated with polydipsia and polyuria in small animal species, and peritonitis has been described as a cause of polyuria/polydipsia in a horse [51–53]. Other clinical signs are likely to predominate in septic conditions, however, and treatment of the primary problem with modalities like intravenous fluid administration may contribute to and therefore obscure the origin of the polyuria. Polyuria in septic conditions may be related to endotoxin-stimulated production of prostaglandin E_2. This eicosanoid has pronounced effects on renal vascular dynamics and water and solute transport in the distal renal tubule and may also inhibit ADH-stimulated water absorption [54]. Polyuria in septic conditions can occur despite significant dehydration but is likely to be a transient phenomenon if the primary condition is successfully addressed [27,52].

Diagnostic approach to the horse with polyuria/polydipsia

Polydipsia can arise from physiologic necessity or as compensation for pathologic polyuria or other disease conditions associated with significant water loss from the body. For this reason, it is of the utmost importance that the clinician thoroughly rules out physiologic causes of polydipsia or pathologic causes of polyuria or water loss before the use of potentially detrimental diagnostic procedures, such as water deprivation testing.

History and physical examination

Initial investigation of the horse with polyuria/polydipsia should include obtaining a detailed history from the owner or trainer with specific emphasis on the duration of the problem; any management changes that occurred in proximity to the onset of the problem; any current and previous medication history; and the composition of the horse's ration, including any dietary supplements. A thorough physical examination should include assessment of hydration status and per rectum examination of the urinary tract. Few clinical abnormalities are likely to be identified in horses with psychogenic polydipsia. Poor body condition, anorexia, and a rough hair coat may suggest chronic renal insufficiency, whereas horses with PPID commonly display hirsutism and may also have abnormal fat deposition and evidence of chronic infections and laminitis [26,55].

Measurement of water intake and urine volume

A concerted effort should be made to confirm the complaint of polydipsia or polyuria and to determine the severity, based on careful and objective measurements of daily water intake and, if necessary, measurement of daily urine volume. Water intake can be determined by periodic measurement of the amount consumed from a single nonautomated water source throughout a 24-hour period [56]. Inaccuracies can result if behavioral tendencies to splash or spill water exist, however. Psychogenic polydipsia and diabetes insipidus often induce extreme polydipsia and the production of voluminous amounts of dilute urine [25,34]. Polydipsia and polyuria associated with renal failure and PPID are usually less pronounced.

Measurement of urine volume is time-consuming and frequently requires cross-tying and close observation of horses throughout the period of attempted urine collection. Several methods of urine collection have been described. These include the use of indwelling Foley catheters in mares and urine collection harnesses specifically designed for mares or geldings [12–16,23,57–59].

Diagnostic procedures

A minimum database for the investigation of polyuria/polydipsia in the horse should include a complete blood cell count, serum biochemistry panel (including blood urea nitrogen [BUN], creatinine, and glucose concentrations), and analysis of a urine sample with determination of specific gravity; reagent strip analysis for glucose, protein, and pigment content; and microscopic examination of urine sediment [33]. Isosthenuria (specific gravity of 1.008–1.014) in the presence of azotemia indicates chronic renal

failure, whereas hyposthenuria (specific gravity <1.007) indicates that renal failure and complete medullary washout are unlikely because renal di-
luting capability is intact [19,26]. Horses may display hyposthenuria rather
than isosthenuria during recovery from acute renal failure; therefore, renal
failure should only be excluded as a differential after appropriate diagnostics [23].

With the exception of hyposthenuria, there are usually no aberrations of
hematologic, biochemical, or urine analyses in horses with psychogenic
polydipsia. Horses with PPID may also show few hematologic and biochemical aberrations, but hyperglycemia, mild neutrophilia, and lymphopenia
may be observed [60]. Glucosuria has also been documented with PPID
but occasionally may indicate non–PPID-associated diabetes mellitus and
possibly renal tubular dysfunction [33]. A suspected diagnosis of PPID
should be confirmed using appropriate endocrine function tests, which generally includes assessment of suppression of serum cortisol concentration in
response to dexamethasone administration (dexamethasone suppression
test) [60,61].

Azotemia in conjunction with isosthenuric urine specific gravity (1.008–
1.014) indicates loss of function of approximately 75% of the nephrons
[28]. Hypercalcemia and hypophosphatemia are also supportive of chronic
renal dysfunction in horses [27,62]. Furthermore, measurement of the fractional clearance of sodium in the urine can be used as an indicator of renal
function. Creatinine and sodium concentrations are measured in concurrently collected urine and serum samples, and the fractional excretion of
sodium is calculated using the equation [15]:

$$FE_{Na}\% = \frac{[Cr]_{plasma}}{[Cr]_{urine}} \times \frac{[Na^+]_{urine}}{[Na^+]_{plasma}} \times 100$$

Documentation of a sodium fractional clearance exceeding 1% is supportive of renal tubular dysfunction or psychogenic salt consumption
[29,63]. Sodium fractional clearance may also approach or exceed 1% in
healthy horses after strenuous exercise, however [64].

Further investigation of renal dysfunction as a possible cause of polyuria/
polydipsia should include transrectal ultrasonographic examination of the
left kidney and urinary tract and transabdominal ultrasonographic imaging
of both kidneys. Abnormal ultrasonographic findings or laboratory findings
suggestive of renal disease warrant more invasive diagnostics, including ultrasound-guided renal biopsy and determination of glomerular filtration
rate [65]. Glomerular filtration rate can decline substantially before the development of azotemia, providing a sensitive indicator of early renal dysfunction [65]. Methods of measuring glomerular filtration rate by means

of radionuclide techniques and various clearance procedures have been described in horses [66–68].

Water deprivation testing

Water deprivation can be used to assess osmoregulatory mechanisms and the ability of the renal tubules to respond to ADH. This method is used to distinguish nephrogenic and central diabetes insipidus from psychogenic polydipsia; therefore, it is usually indicated in animals displaying hyposthenuria [19,20]. Water deprivation testing should not be performed in horses that are azotemic or dehydrated, and other pathologic causes of polydipsia/polyuria should be ruled out in advance [21,30]. In healthy animals, water deprivation prompts an increase in plasma osmolality that provokes ADH release, with a subsequent increase in urine specific gravity and osmolality. The physiologic responses of healthy horses to water deprivation have been thoroughly described, and after 48 hours of water deprivation, healthy horses generate urine specific gravity values greater than 1.040 and as high as 1.054 [69,70].

A water deprivation test is commenced after preliminary urine and blood samples are obtained. The bladder is emptied and a baseline body weight is obtained before the horse is confined without access to water. Body weight, urine specific gravity, and, potentially, BUN concentration are measured periodically, typically every 6 hours to every 12 hours. More frequent clinical monitoring of hydration status is also important to decrease the risk for developing profound dehydration [68]. An appropriate response to water deprivation is an increase in urine specific gravity to greater than 1.025 after 24 hours or once 5% of body weight has been lost [27]. The test should be terminated once an appropriate urine specific gravity is achieved, if the horse loses 5% of its body weight, or if dehydration or azotemia occurs [68].

Horses with psychogenic polydipsia are expected to display an appropriate increase in urine specific gravity in response to water deprivation. However, excessive water consumption for several weeks or more creates a reduction in medullary tonicity subsequently, impairing renal concentrating ability [28]. Therefore, horses with long-standing psychogenic polydipsia may not be capable of increasing urine concentration to greater than a specific gravity of 1.020 during abrupt water deprivation. In such cases, modified water deprivation testing involving restriction of water intake to 40 mL/kg of body weight per day for 3 to 4 days with frequent assessment of hydration status and urine specific gravity should allow re-establishment of medullary hypertonicity and production of urine with a specific gravity exceeding 1.025 by the end of the testing period [26,27]. An intermediate response to abrupt or modified water deprivation (urine specific gravity > 1.008 and < 1.020) may also be consistent with partial neurogenic diabetes insipidus or renal insufficiency, and appropriate diagnostics should be pursued to rule these conditions out [19,30]. If complete central or nephrogenic diabetes insipidus is present, horses continue to produce dilute urine (specific gravity <1.008), with a progressive loss of body weight [30]. Distinguishing these two conditions requires measurement of endogenous ADH concentration or assessing the response to exogenous ADH response as described here [30].

Measurement of plasma antidiuretic hormone and response to exogenous antidiuretic hormone or antidiuretic hormone analogues

Measurement of plasma ADH concentration and assessment of the response to exogenously administered ADH or an ADH analogue are usually reserved for the diagnosis of central or nephrogenic diabetes insipidus, and therefore rarely indicated in horses [34,42,43].

Measurement of plasma ADH concentration during water deprivation testing can be used to distinguish the cause of disturbed water conservation. An elevation of plasma ADH concentration without a corresponding increase in urine specific gravity is supportive of nephrogenic diabetes insipidus, whereas a minimal increase in plasma ADH concentration is supportive of central diabetes insipidus. Similarly, endogenous ADH concentration can be measured before and 30 minutes after administration of 7.5% sodium chloride solution (1–2 mL/kg) [34,71]. Intravenous infusion of hypertonic saline increases plasma osmolality and triggers ADH release [21]. If psychogenic polydipsia is the cause of the polyuria, affected horses should have an increase in plasma ADH concentration in response to hypertonic saline infusion. Similarly, plasma ADH concentration should also increase with nephrogenic diabetes insipidus but not with central diabetes insipidus [68]. Unfortunately, clinical use of this test is currently limited because of a lack of commercially available procedures for measuring equine plasma ADH concentration.

The ability of the renal tubules to respond to ADH can be assessed by means of the administration of aqueous synthetic vasopressin or desmopressin acetate (DDAVP), a potent synthetic analogue, with subsequent monitoring of urine specific gravity [30]. Aqueous synthetic vasopressin (20-U/mL formulation) can be administered intramuscularly (0.25–0.5 U/kg) or as an intravenous infusion (5 U in 5% dextrose [1 L] administered at a rate of 2.5 mU/kg over 60 minutes) [30]. Urine specific gravity is expected to increase to 1.020 or higher within 60 to 90 minutes after administration unless nephrogenic diabetes insipidus is present [30]. DDAVP has greater antidiuretic potency compared with synthetic aqueous vasopressin, with minimal pressor action and less impact on visceral smooth muscle [68]. To determine renal concentrating ability in the horse, urine specific gravity and plasma osmolality can be measured every 2 hours after the administration of DDAVP [27,68]. The nasal spray formulation (DDAVP, 0.1 mg/mL) can be diluted in sterile water, and 0.05 μg/kg can be administered intravenously for this purpose [68]. An increase in urine specific gravity to 1.025 or greater within 2 hours after administration would be considered consistent with central diabetes insipidus, whereas a lack of response is consistent with nephrogenic diabetes insipidus if medullary washout has been accounted for [28,42,43,68].

Management of polyuria and polydipsia

Management of polyuria and polydipsia varies somewhat depending on the underlying cause. Psychogenic polydipsia should be addressed by altering the horse's management and environment to relieve boredom [26,27]. Helpful strategies may include increased exercise or turnout time, increased frequency of meals, constant availability of roughage, or provision of a companion. Provision of drinking water should be limited to a volume appropriate for estimated requirements based on environmental factors and workload. Water restriction should only be practiced once underlying renal disease or metabolic conditions have been definitively ruled out, however [72]. Psychogenic salt ingestion should be addressed by preventing access to free-choice mineral sources and top-dressing feed to meet estimated requirements.

Horse with renal dysfunction or nephrogenic or central diabetes insipidus should have unrestricted access to fresh water to avoid dehydration or exacerbation of renal dysfunction. Electrolyte and mineral supplementation may be required to compensate for urinary losses, although calcium intake should be limited in horses with renal failure to avoid exacerbating hypercalcemia. Periodic monitoring of serum electrolyte, BUN, and creatinine concentrations should be performed, and a highly palatable high-energy diet should be provided. Restriction of sodium and water intake and treatment with thiazide diuretics, prostaglandin inhibitors, or amiloride (a sodium channel blocker) may decrease the immensity of polyuria associated with nephrogenic diabetes insipidus in human beings and other animals, but their effects have not been assessed in horses [72,73]. Specific treatment of central diabetes insipidus using exogenous vasopressin or desmopressin is performed successfully in small animal species but has not been described in the horse [40,41]. Treatment of horses would likely be cost-prohibitive, and efficacy is currently unknown.

Polyuria in horses with PPID may respond to treatment with dopamine agonists, including bromocriptine or pergolide [26]. Trilostane, a competitive inhibitor of 3-β hydroxysteroid dehydrogenase, which is used to treat canine pituitary-dependent hyperadrenocorticism, has also been reported to improve polyuria and polydipsia and other clinical signs of PPID in affected horses [36].

References

[1] Groenendyk S, English PB, Abetz I. External balance of water and electrolytes in the horse. Equine Vet J 1988;20(3):189–93.

[2] Cymbaluk NF. Water balance of horses fed various diets. Equine Pract 1989;11(1):19–24.

[3] Tasker JB. Fluid and electrolyte studies in the horse. III. Intake and output of water, sodium and potassium in normal horses. Cornell Vet 1967;57:649–57.

[4] Lewis D. Water, energy, protein, carbohydrates, and fats for horses. In: Lewis D, editor. Equine clinical nutrition—feeding and care. Media (PA): Williams and Wilkins; 1995. p. 3–24.

[5] Knottenbelt DC. Polyuria-polydipsia in the horse. Equine Vet Educ 2000;12(4):179–86.

[6] McCutcheon LJ, Geor RJ. Sweat fluid and ion losses in horses during training and competition in cool vs. hot ambient conditions: implications for ion supplementation. Equine Vet J 1996;22(Suppl):54–62.

[7] Sufit E, Houpt KA, Sweeting M. Physiological stimuli of thirst and drinking patterns in ponies. Equine Vet J 1985;17(1):12–6.

[8] Pearson RA, Cuddeford D, Archibald RF, et al. Digestibility of diets containing different proportions of alfalfa and oat straw in Thoroughbreds, Shetland Ponies, Highland Ponies and Donkeys. Proc Europaische Konferenz über die Ernahrung des Pferdes Hannover; 1992. p. 153–7.

[9] Houpt KA. Thirst in horses: the physiological and psychological causes. Equine Pract 1987; 9:28–30.

[10] Houpt KA, Eggleston A, Kunkle K, et al. Effect of water restriction on equine behaviour and physiology. Equine Vet J 2000;32(4):341–4.

[11] Rawlings CA, Bisgard GE. Renal clearance and excretion of endogenous substances in the small pony. Am J Vet Res 1975;36(1):45–8.

[12] Kohn CW, Strasser SL. 24-Hour renal clearance and excretion of endogenous substances in the mare. Am J Vet Res 1986;47(6):1332–7.

[13] Morris DD, Divers TJ, Whitlock RH. Renal clearance and fractional excretion of electrolytes over a 24-hour period in horses. Am J Vet Res 1984;45(11):2431–5.

[14] Rumbaugh GE, Carlson GP, Harrold D. Urinary production in the healthy horse and in horses deprived of feed and water. Am J Vet Res 1982;43(4):735–7.

[15] McKenzie EC, Valberg SJ, Godden SM, et al. Comparison of volumetric urine collection versus single sample urine collection in horses consuming diets varying in cation-anion balance. Am J Vet Res 2003;64(3):284–91.

[16] Brewer BD, Clement SF, Lotz WS, et al. Renal clearance, urinary excretion of endogenous substances and urinary diagnostic indices in healthy neonatal foals. J Vet Intern Med 1991; 5(1):28–33.

[17] Edwards DJ, Brownlow MA, Hutchins DR. Indices of renal function; values in eight normal foals from birth to 56 days. Aust Vet J 1990;67(6):251–4.

[18] Martin RG, McMeniman NP, Dowsett KF. Milk and water intakes of foals sucking grazing mares. Equine Vet J 1992;24(4):295–9.

[19] Hughes D. Polyuria and polydipsia. Compend Cont Educ Pract Vet 1992;14(9):1161–75.

[20] Jane JA, Vance ML, Laws ER. Neurogenic diabetes insipidus. Pituitary 2006;9(4):327–9.

[21] Grauer GF. The differential diagnosis of polyuric-polydipsic diseases. Compend Contin Educ Pract Vet 1981;3(12):1079–84.

[22] Nichols R. Polyuria and polydipsia. Diagnostic approach and problems associated with patient evaluation. Vet Clin North Am Small Anim Pract 2001;31(5):833–44.

[23] Schott HC. Polyuria and polydipsia. In: Reed SM, Bayly WM, editors. Equine internal medicine. Philadelphia: WB Saunders; 1998. p. 895–901.

[24] Carlson GP. Fluid and electrolyte dynamics in the horse. In: Proc Annu Vet Med Forum Am Coll Vet Intern Med San Diego:1987;5:7–29.

[25] Browning AP. Polydipsia and polyuria in two horses caused by psychogenic polydipsia. Equine Vet Educ 2000;12(4):175–8.

[26] Brown CM. Polyuria. In: Robinson NE, editor. Current therapy in equine medicine 4. Philadelphia: WB Saunders; 1997. p. 486–8.

[27] Knottenbelt DC. Differential diagnosis of polyuria/polydipsia. In: Robinson NE, editor. Current therapy in equine medicine 5. Philadelphia: WB Saunders; 2003. p. 828–31.

[28] Whitlock RH. Polyuria. In: Robinson NE, editor. Current therapy in equine medicine 3. Philadelphia: WB Saunders; 1992. p. 620–2.

[29] Buntain BJ, Coffman JR. Polyuria and polydipsia in a horse induced by psychogenic salt consumption. Equine Vet J 1981;13(4):266–8.

[30] Kohn CW, Hansen B. Polyuria and polydipsia. In: Reed SM, Bayly WM, Sellon DC, editors. Equine internal medicine. 2nd edition. St Louis (MO): Saunders; 2004. p. 114–20.

[31] Lewis LD. Minerals for horses. In: Equine clinical nutrition—feeding and care. Media (PA): Williams and Wilkins; 1995. p. 35.

[32] Schryver HF, Parker MT, Daniluk PD, et al. Salt consumption and the effect of salt on mineral metabolism in horses. Cornell Vet 1987;77(2):122–31.

[33] Koterba AM, Coffman JR. Acute and chronic renal disease in the horse. Compend Contin Educ Pract Vet 1981;12(3):S461–9.

[34] Schott HC, Bayly WM, Reed SM, et al. Nephrogenic diabetes insipidus in sibling colts. J Vet Intern Med 1993;7(2):68–72.

[35] Thurmon JC, Steffey EP, Zinkl JG, et al. Xylazine causes transient dose-related hyperglycemia and increased urine volumes in mares. Am J Vet Res 1984;45(2):224–7.

[36] McGowan CM, Neiger R. Efficacy of trilostane for the treatment of equine Cushing's syndrome. Equine Vet J 2003;35(4):414–8.

[37] Hillyer MH, Taylor FGR, Mair TS. Diagnosis of hyperadrenocorticism in the horse. Equine Vet Educ 1992;4:131–4.

[38] Meyer TW, Scholey JW, Brenner BM. Nephron adaptation to renal injury. In: Brenner BM, Rector FC, editors. The kidney. 4th edition. Philadelphia: WB Saunders; 1991. p. 1871–908.

[39] Ehnen SJ, Divers TJ, Gillette D, et al. Obstructive nephrolithiasis and ureterolithiasis associated with chronic renal failure in horses: eight cases (1981–1987). J Am Vet Med Assoc 1990;197(2):249–53.

[40] Aroch I, Mazaki-Tovi M, Shemesh O, et al. Central diabetes insipidus in five cats: clinical presentation, diagnosis and oral desmopressin therapy. J Feline Med Surg 2005;7(6):333–9.

[41] Harb MF, Nelson RW, Feldman EC, et al. Central diabetes insipidus in dogs: 20 cases (1986–1995). J Am Vet Med Assoc 1996;209(11):1884–8.

[42] Breukink HJ, Van Wegen P, Schotman AJH. Idiopathic diabetes insipidus in a Welsh Pony. Equine Vet J 1983;15(3):284–7.

[43] Filar J, Ziolo T, Szalecki J. Diabetes insipidus in the course of encephalitis in the horse. Med Weter 1971;27:205–7.

[44] Ruoff WW, Baker DC, Morgan SJ. Type II diabetes mellitus in a horse. Equine Vet J 1986; 18(2):143–4.

[45] Jeffrey JR. Diabetes mellitus secondary to chronic pancreatitis in a pony. J Am Vet Med Assoc 1969;153(9):1168–75.

[46] Muylle E, Van Den Hende C, Deprez P, et al. Non-insulin dependent diabetes mellitus in a horse. Equine Vet J 1986;18(2):145–6.

[47] Johnson PJ, Scotty NC, Wiedmeyer C, et al. Diabetes mellitus in a domesticated Spanish mustang. J Am Vet Med Assoc 2005;226(4):584–8.

[48] McCoy DJ. Diabetes mellitus associated with bilateral granulosa cell tumors in a mare. J Am Vet Med Assoc 1986;188(7):733–5.

[49] Ryu SH, Kim BS, Lee CW, et al. Glucocorticoid-induced laminitis with hepatopathy in a Thoroughbred filly. J Vet Sci 2004;5(3):271–4.

[50] Cohen ND, Carter GK. Steroid hepatopathy in a horse with glucocorticoid-induced hyperadrenocorticism. J Am Vet Med Assoc 1992;200(11):1682–4.

[51] Hardy RM, Osborne CA. Canine pyometra: pathophysiology, diagnosis and treatment of uterine and extrauterine lesions. J Am Anim Hosp Assoc 1974;10:245–68.

[52] Asheim A. Pathogenesis of renal damage and polydipsia in dogs with pyometra. J Am Vet Med Assoc 1965;147(7):736–45.

[53] Traver DS, Moore JN, Coffman JR, et al. Peritonitis in a horse: a cause of acute abdominal distress and polyuria-polydipsia. J Equine Med Surg 1977;1:36–9.

[54] Breyer MD, Breyer RM. Prostaglandin E receptors and the kidney. Am J Physiol Renal Physiol 2000;279(1):F12–23.

[55] Schott HC. Pituitary pars intermedia dysfunction: equine Cushing's disease. Vet Clin North Am Equine Pract 2002;18(2):237–70.

[56] Sneddon JC, Colyn P. A practical system for measuring water intake in stabled horses. Equine Vet Sci 1991;11:141.

[57] van den Berg IS. Modified apparatus for collection of free-flow urine from mares. J S Afr Vet Assoc 1996;67(4):214–6.

[58] Tasker JB. Fluid and electrolyte studies in the horse. II. An apparatus for the collection of total daily urine and feces from horses. Cornell Vet 1966;56(1):77–84.

[59] Harris P. Collection of urine. Equine Vet J 1988;20(2):86–8.

[60] Dybdal NO. Endocrine disorders. In: Smith BP, editor. Large animal internal medicine, 3rd edition. St. Louis (MO); 2002. p. 1233–41.

[61] Dybdal NO, Hargreaves KM, Madigan JE, et al. Diagnostic testing for pituitary pars intermedia dysfunction in horses. J Am Vet Med Assoc 1994;204(4):627–32.

[62] Tennant B, Bettleheim P, Kaneko JJ. Paradoxic hypercalcemia and hypophosphatemia associated with chronic renal failure in horses. J Am Vet Med Assoc 1982;180(6):630–4.

[63] Grossman BS, Brobst DF, Kramer JW, et al. Urinary indices for differentiation of prerenal azotemia and renal azotemia in horses. J Am Vet Med Assoc 1982;180(3):284–8.

[64] Cohen ND, Roussel AJ, Lumsden JH, et al. Alterations of fluid and electrolyte balance in Thoroughbred racehorses following strenuous exercise during training. Can J Vet Res 1993;57:9–13.

[65] Pringle J. Pathophysiology and diagnosis of urinary disease. In: Kobluck CN, Ames TR, Geor RJ, editors. The horse: diseases and clinical management. Philadelphia: WB Saunders; 1995. p. 575–81.

[66] Matthews HK, Andrews FM, Daniel GB, et al. Comparison of standard and radionuclide methods for measurement of glomerular filtration rate and effective renal blood flow in female horses. Am J Vet Res 1992;53(9):1612–6.

[67] Brewer BD, Clement SF, Lotz WS, et al. A comparison of inulin, para-aminohippuric acid, and endogenous creatinine clearances as measures of renal function in neonatal foals. J Vet Intern Med 1990;4(6):301–5.

[68] Schott HC. Examination of the urinary system. In: Reed SM, Bayly WM, Sellon DC, editors. Equine internal medicine. 2nd edition. St Louis (MO): Saunders; 2004. p. 1200–20.

[69] Brobst DF, Bayly WM. Responses of horses to a water deprivation test. Equine Vet Sci 1982; 2:51–6.

[70] Genetzky RM, Loparco FV, Ledet AE. Clinical pathologic alterations in horses during a water deprivation test. Am J Vet Res 1987;48(6):1007–11.

[71] Irvine CHG, Alexander SL, Donald RA. Effect of an osmotic stimulus on the secretion of arginine vasopressin and adrenocorticotropin in the horse. Endocrinology 1989;124(6): 3102–8.

[72] Schott HC. Polyuria and polydipsia. In: Smith BP, editor. Equine internal medicine. 3rd edition. St Louis (MO): Mosby; 2002. p. 845–7.

[73] Takemura N. Successful long-term treatment of congenital nephrogenic diabetes insipidus in a dog. J Small Anim Pract 1998;39(12):592–4.

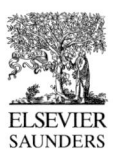

ELSEVIER
SAUNDERS

VETERINARY
CLINICS
Equine Practice

Vet Clin Equine 23 (2007) 655–675

Hematuria and Pigmenturia of Horses

John Schumacher, DVM, MS

*Department of Clinical Sciences, College of Veterinary Medicine,
Auburn University, Auburn, AL 36849, USA*

This article discusses hematuria and pigmenturia of horses. Equine urine is normally straw colored. Discolored urine can be caused by contamination with red blood cells, hemoglobin, myoglobin, oxidizing agents normally found in urine, and plant-derived pigments.

Determining the cause of urine discoloration

The presence of red or brown discoloration of freshly voided urine (Fig. 1) indicates hematuria or pigmenturia (hemoglobin, myoglobin, or plant-derived pigments). Hematuria is obvious if the urine is so heavily contaminated with blood that blood clots are voided during urination; however, when urine is only blood tinged, distinguishing hematuria from hemoglobinuria or myoglobinuria may require urinalysis and biochemical analysis of serum. To establish that red discoloration of urine is caused by red blood cells, urine can be centrifuged to observe a layer of red blood cells covered by clear urine. Urine remains discolored after centrifugation if hemoglobin, myoglobin, or a plant pigment has caused the discoloration. An abundance of red blood cells found during microscopic examination of discolored urine suggests hematuria, whereas absence of red blood cells suggests pigmenturia. Red blood cells may rupture if examination of urine, especially if it is dilute, is delayed (for as little as 1–2 hours), resulting in false hemoglobinuria. In this case, red blood cell ghosts may be seen during microscopic examination of sediment. Clinical signs of myopathy and markedly increased serum creatine kinase (CK) activity indicate myoglobinuria as a cause of urine discoloration. Activity of CK is increased to at least several thousand U/L when significant muscle injury has occurred [1]. Hemoglobinuria after systemic hemolysis is associated with pink to red discolored serum, whereas the serum of horses having myoglobinuria is clear because this

E-mail address: schumjo@vetmed.auburn.edu

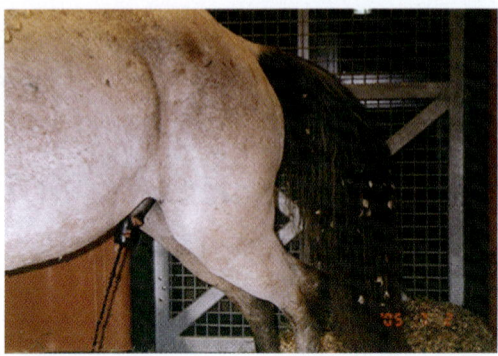

Fig. 1. The presence of red or brown discoloration of freshly voided urine indicates hematuria or the presence of pigments, such as hemoglobin, myoglobin, or plant-derived pigments.

pigment is rapidly cleared from the serum. When there is hemolysis, plasma is discolored even before hemoglobin is in a high enough concentration to result in hemoglobinuria [2]. Hematuria, hemoglobinuria, and myoglobinuria all result in a positive reagent strip analysis. A negative reagent strip analysis of red or brown urine suggests that plant-derived pigments are the cause of discoloration. A false-positive reagent strip analysis can sometimes occur when bacteria are present in the urine.

Oxidizing agents normally found in urine cause the normal yellow color of equine urine to darken on standing [3]. Normal equine urine also may contain pigments that can stain bedding red or cause urine to turn red after exposure to air or after contact with snow. Horse owners may report erroneously that their horse has voided bloody urine if they are unaware that equine urine may change color after urination.

Oxidizing agents called pyrocatechins are claimed to be the cause of the red or brown color imparted to urine on standing [3]. Red urine associated with feeding white clover to horses is claimed to be caused by oxidative breakdown products of tryptophan [4]. Deer grazing red clover voided urine normal in color that turned scarlet red 1 hour after exposure to air [5]. Although the pigments were found not to be tryptophan derivatives, they were not identified. A phenolic compound was suspected to be the cause of a change in urine color to orange red that occurred 5 minutes after micturition in dairy cattle [6]. Administration of drugs such as rifampin, phenothiazine, and nitazoxanide can cause a bright orange or red discoloration of urine. Doxycycline can change the color of urine to dark brown or black. Urine of some horses is naturally orange in color.

Hematuria

Evaluation of horses with hematuria

Blood can mix with urine in the kidney, ureter, bladder, urethra, or reproductive tract. Initial evaluation of horses with hematuria should include palpation per rectum of the accessible portion of the urinary tract; urinalysis; urine culture; and endoscopic examination of the urethra, bladder, and ureteral orifices. For mares, examination of the reproductive system should also be performed.

Urinalysis

Urinalysis may not be possible if the urine contains a large quantity of blood. Urine collected during midstream and end-stream urination is most desirable for cytologic examination because nondiagnostic cellular debris is flushed before collection. Cells associated with lower urinary tract disease settle out in the bladder and are more likely to be found in an end-stream sample. Cells indicative of upper urinary tract disease are most likely to be found on a midstream sample. If urine cannot be examined within 30 minutes, it should be refrigerated to avoid changes in pH, cellular degeneration, and bacterial growth. After urine is observed for gross appearance, specific gravity, and reagent strip reactions, it is centrifuged for microscopic examination of sediment. When urine is collected by catheterization, hematuria is usually defined as more than 5 red blood cells per high-powered field and pyuria is usually defined as a white blood cell count of at least 10 white blood cells/mm^3, or more than 5 white blood cells per high-powered field [7]. When urine is collected during urination, up to 8 red and white blood cells per high-powered field are considered normal [7].

Quantitative urine culture

Failure to find bacteria or increased numbers of white blood cells during light microscopy does not rule out bacterial infection of the urinary tract [8]. When urinary tract infection is suspected as a cause of hematuria, quantitative urine culture should be performed. Urine submitted for enumeration of pathogenic bacteria should be collected by catheterization rather than during urination to avoid contamination of the sample with bacteria that normally reside in the distal portion of the urethra. Recovery of more than 10,000 colony-forming units per milliliter of urine collected by catheterization indicates a urinary tract infection, but contamination of the catheter with bacteria from the perineum, vestibule, or distal portion of the urethra might account for a quantitative bacterial culture indicative of infection [8].

Complete blood cell count and serum biochemistries

Because some horses with hematuria become anemic and hypoproteinemic, a complete blood cell count and serum protein concentration should be performed. Evaluation of serum concentrations of blood urea nitrogen, creatinine, and electrolytes may help to determine if the horse has renal disease. Coagulation tests for horses with hematuria should be considered if the cause of hematuria is not obvious after physical, ultrasonographic, endoscopic, or clinicopathologic examination. For horses fed alfalfa hay that have hematuria and clinical signs compatible with blister beetle toxicosis, urine should be submitted to a diagnostic laboratory for detection of cantharidin.

Endoscopy

Endoscopy is useful in the diagnosis of cystitis, urinary calculi, urethral rents, renal hemorrhage, and cystic neoplasia. Endoscopy of the male urinary tract is performed using a sterile 100-cm or longer flexible endoscope with a diameter no larger than 12 mm. The endoscope can be sterilized according to the manufacturer's recommendations or with a glutaraldehyde-based product and then rinsed with sterile water [9]. The accessory channel should also be lavaged with disinfectant and rinsed with sterile water. Male horses usually must be sedated for endoscopic examination of the urinary tract. Using endoscopy, urine can be collected from the bladder or ureters to locate the site of hemorrhage more accurately and to assess functioning of each kidney. To collect urine from a ureter, polyethylene tubing, passed through the accessory channel of the endoscope, is inserted into a ureteral orifice (Fig. 2). The ureteral openings are observed in the dorsal aspect of the trigone region at the 10 and 2 o'clock positions. The ureteral openings can be found by watching for dilation of the openings as a spurt of urine is discharged. Urine is discharged from the ureters in spurts approximately once every minute (Fig. 3). Placement of a ureteral catheter in the mare without the aid of an endoscope has been described [10].

Ultrasonography

Ultrasonographic examination of the kidneys or a renal biopsy should be considered if lesions of the lower urinary tract are unlikely based on history,

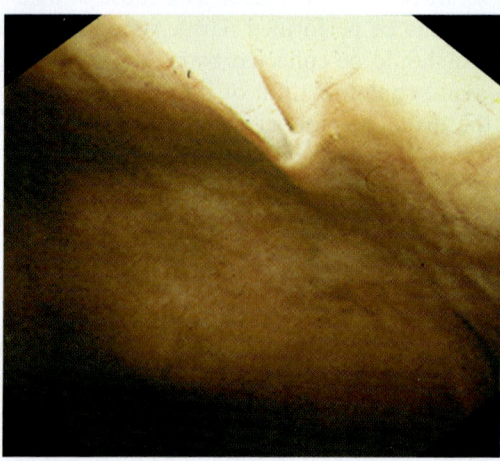

Fig. 2. Using endoscopy, urine can be collected from the bladder or ureters to locate the site of hemorrhage more accurately and to assess functioning of each kidney. To collect urine from a ureter, polyethylene tubing, passed through the accessory channel of the endoscope, is inserted into a ureteral orifice.

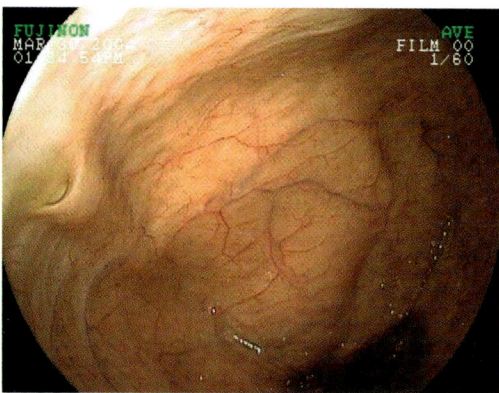

Fig. 3. The ureteral openings are observed in the dorsal aspect of the trigone region at the 10 and 2 o'clock positions. The ureteral openings can be found by watching for dilation of the openings as a spurt of urine is discharged.

clinical signs, or initial examination or if blood is seen emanating from a ureteral orifice during endoscopy (Fig. 4). Percutaneous ultrasonographic examination of the kidneys is performed using a real-time B-mode ultrasound scanner with a 3- to 3.5-MHz sector transducer (5 MHz for foals). The right kidney is usually imaged ventral to the transverse processes at the 14th to 16th intercostal spaces, and the left kidney is usually imaged at the 17th intercostal space and paralumbar fossa in a space between horizontal parallel lines drawn from the tuber coxae and tuber ischii [11].

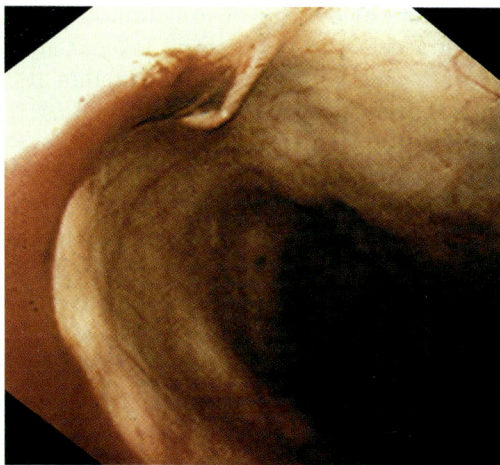

Fig. 4. If blood is seen emanating from a ureteral orifice during endoscopy, ultrasonography of that kidney is indicated.

Renal biopsy

Biopsy of the kidney may provide the diagnosis if hematuria is renal in origin. Renal biopsy is a safe procedure, particularly if ultrasonography is used to aid in the procedure. A hemostatic profile should be performed before a kidney is biopsied because evidence of a coagulopathy is a contraindication for performing the procedure [12]. The horse should be restrained adequately during renal biopsy because movement during the procedure can result in laceration of the kidney or spleen. The kidney is usually biopsied with a Franklin-modified or Tru-Cut–style biopsy needle. The kidney can be blindly biopsied percutaneously, but ultrasonographic guidance of the biopsy needle allows accurate identification of the site for biopsy and increases the safety of the technique by identifying large blood vessels to be avoided with the biopsy instrument. Using ultrasonography, the depth of the kidney can be measured. Marking the needle for depth of penetration can increase the likelihood of obtaining renal cortex and medulla in the sample. Biopsy of the right kidney is usually performed at the 15th–17th intercostal spaces, on or above a line connecting the tuber coxae to the point of the shoulder, with the needle inserted perpendicular to the body wall [13]. For most horses, the needle is advanced slightly more than 3 cm to contact the right kidney. The left kidney is biopsied through the left flank near a line connecting the tuber coxae to the point of the shoulder. The depth of penetration to reach the left kidney varies but is often approximately 7 cm. For some horses, the spleen must be penetrated to biopsy the left kidney [13].

Conditions causing hematuria

Urethral rents

Hematuria that occurs at the end of urination in geldings is typical of a condition in which a defect in the urethral mucosa allows blood within the corpus spongiosum penis (CSP) to enter the urethra at the end of urination [14–16]. Urethral rents occur on the convex surface of the urethra of male horses at the level of the ischial arch (Fig. 5). The same defect does not cause hematuria in stallions but, instead, is associated with hemospermia. Some horses with urethral rents display signs of dysuria (eg, tenesmus, grunting). Hemorrhage through the rent into the urethral lumen occurs when pressure within the CSP increases at the end of urination or during ejaculation. The bulbospongiosus muscle causes this increase in pressure as it contracts to expel the contents of the urethra at the end of urination or during ejaculation [17]. The reason for the difference in clinical signs between stallions and geldings is because the CSP of geldings reaches a higher pressure during urination than does the CSP of stallions [18]. The CSP of geldings is smaller that of stallions, and pressure applied to a smaller space creates more pressure within that space than pressure applied to a larger space.

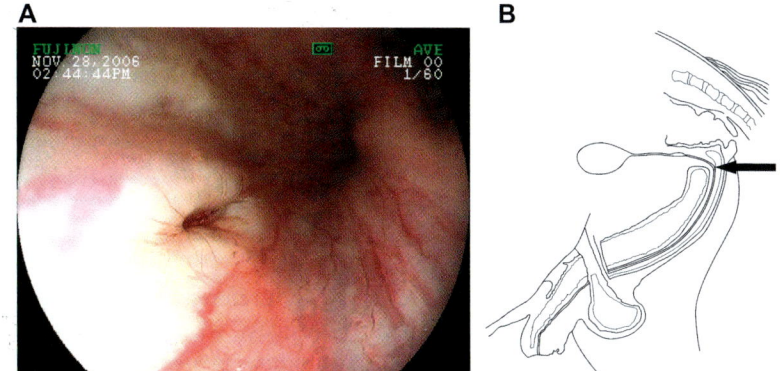

Fig. 5. (*A, B*) Urethra rents invariably occur on the convex surface of the urethra of male horses at the level of the ischial arch (*arrow in B*).

Endoscopic examination of the urethra is required for diagnosis of a urethral rent. A 5- to 10-mm linear defect can be identified on the convex surface of the urethra, distal to the openings of the bulbourethral glands, near the level of the ischial arch. The cause of urethral rents is not known, but because the defect is invariably found on the convex surface of the urethra at the level of the ischial arch, the tunica albuginea of the CSP in this location may be subject to increased pressure during urination [18].

Urethral rents often heal without treatment [19], but surgical treatment may speed recovery. Affected geldings (or stallions) can be treated by means of a temporary ischial urethrotomy or by an ischial incision that extends into the CSP but does not enter the lumen of the urethra [15,20]. Surgery is performed with the horse standing and sedated after administration of epidural anesthesia or local anesthesia. After an endoscope or catheter is inserted into the urethra and advanced proximal to the defect to facilitate recognition of the urethra during surgery, an 8-cm vertical cutaneous incision is created on the perineal raphe and centered on the ischial arch. The incision is extended through the retractor penis and bulbospongiosus muscles and the tunica albuginea that surrounds the CSP. An incision into the urethral lumen is not necessary to promote healing of the rent. The incision heals by second intention within approximately 3 weeks. Because the "pressure valve" created by the ischial incision reduces pressure within the CSP, hematuria is not observed after surgery. Horses bleed from the perineal wound, however, especially at the end of urination [15].

Incising the CSP encourages blood within the CSP to exit the subischial incision rather than the urethral rent during contraction of the bulbospongiosus muscle at the end of urination, thereby allowing the rent to heal [15]. Incising the CSP without entering the urethra seems to be effective in eliminating hematuria caused by urethral rents and might reduce the risk for urethral fistulas or strictures.

Urethritis

Although urethritis may be an actual cause of hematuria or hemospermia, a diagnosis of urethritis as a cause of hematuria could be an erroneous interpretation of the endoscopic appearance of the normal male urethra [21]. When the urethra dilates with air during endoscopic examination, the vasculature and cavernosal spaces surrounding the urethra become prominent in the proximal portion of the urethra (Fig. 6) [22]. The prominent vasculature and cavernosal spaces may be mistaken as inflammation or even hemorrhage.

Larvae of *Draschia* and *Habronema* spp have preferential sites for development in moist areas, such as the urethral process, where they are deposited by flies attracted to moisture. A granuloma involving the urethral process, caused by infestation of these larvae, can be a cause of hematuria in horses [23]. Erosion of the CSP by the granuloma results in hemorrhage when pressure within the CSP increases at the end of urination. Horses affected by habronemiasis are treated with topically or systemically administered corticosteroids to reduce the hypersensitivity reaction to the larvae and by systemic or topical administration of organophosphates to kill the larvae. The anthelmintic ivermectin may also kill *Habronema* larvae [24,25]. When medical treatment is unsuccessful, amputation of the urethral process usually is effective treatment of horses affected with habronemiasis of the urethral process [26].

Bacterial cystitis

Cystitis is a rare cause of hematuria in horses. Cystitis in the horse is usually secondary to urine retention caused by paresis or paralysis of the bladder or by a urocystolith [16,27]. Vaginitis and repeated or prolonged indwelling catheterization are other predisposing causes of bacterial cystitis.

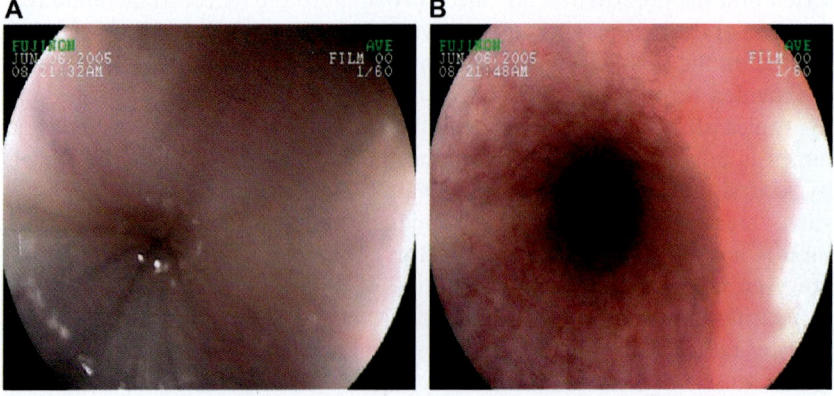

Fig. 6. (*A*) On the left, the urethra of a male horse is seen during endoscopic examination before it has been dilated with air. (*B*) Urethra on the right has been dilated with air, making the vasculature and cavernosal spaces beneath the mucosa prominent.

Primary or idiopathic cystitis in the horse is rare. In addition to hematuria, other clinical signs of cystitis include dysuria and frequent urination (ie, pollakiuria). The bladder usually feels normal during palpation per rectum, but thickening and erosions of the bladder mucosa may be seen during cystoscopy.

For horses with cystitis, bacterial culture of urine and antimicrobial sensitivity testing of cultured bacteria are indicated. Affected horses should be treated with an antimicrobial drug excreted in high concentration in urine, such as penicillin, gentamicin, amikacin, enrofloxacin, or trimethoprim-sulfa, if microbes cultured from urine are sensitive to the drug. For horses with cystitis secondary to other conditions, correction of the inciting disease (eg, urolithiasis), if possible, and antimicrobial therapy are indicated.

Urolithiasis

Hematuria observed after exercise, the most common clinical sign displayed by horses affected with a cystic calculus, is virtually pathognomonic for the condition [16,28]. Even though hematuria is not a clinical sign of most horses affected with nephrolithiasis or ureterolithiasis [29–32], exercise-induced hematuria has also been observed in horses with nephrolithiasis [28,33]. Whereas hemorrhage associated with urethral rents occurs immediately after urination, hematuria caused by cystic calculi is likely to be more pronounced near the end of urination [15,28].

Other clinical signs of cystic or urethral calculi include pollakiuria, dribbling of urine, dysuria, and prolonged periods of penile protrusion [34–36]. The hind limbs are often urine or blood stained. A cystic calculus may cause a stilted hind limb gait. These signs may help to distinguish horses with a cystic calculus from horses with a urethral rent because a urethral rent usually causes no signs of pain.

Cystic uroliths are usually singular, round, or egg-shaped. They may be white, smooth, and hard, but most are yellow green in color and rough. Those with a rough surface are often imbedded in mucosa and tend to be larger and more friable than smooth stones (Fig. 7) [35,37]. Cystic uroliths are found more frequently in male horses than in mares.

The presence of a cystic calculus can usually be confirmed by palpation of the bladder per rectum or by observing the calculus during endoscopic examination of the bladder. The pelvic portion of the urethra should be palpated, in addition to the bladder, so that a calculus in this location is not overlooked. A cystic calculus is more likely to be detected if only the hand and wrist are inserted into the rectum to palpate the bladder [16]. A urethral calculus can be identified using ultrasonography and endoscopy, during passage of a urinary catheter, or by careful palpation of the urethra.

The following factors should be considered when choosing the method of removal of a cystic urolith: size and texture of the urolith, anesthetic risks, and economic constraints. Cystic uroliths can be removed by means of standing ischial urethrotomy, celiocystotomy, or pararectal cystotomy (ie,

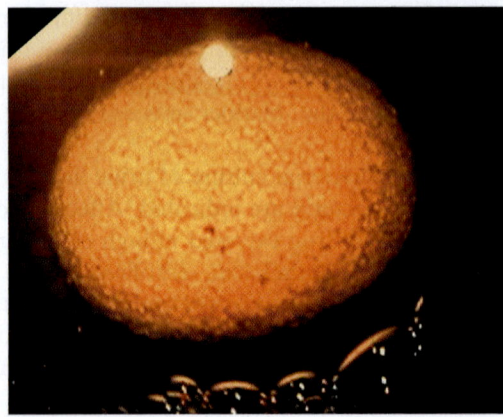

Fig. 7. Most bladder stones are yellow green in color and rough. Those with a rough surface are often imbedded in mucosa and tend to be larger and more friable.

Gokel's operation). Sometimes, a urolith must be fragmented (ie, litho-tripsy) before it can be removed by urethrotomy. To remove a calculus from any area of the urethra, the horse can be anesthetized or the procedure can be performed with the horse standing using chemical restraint and local or regional anesthesia. Urethral incisions are usually left unsutured to heal as an open wound. Cystic, ureteral, and urethral uroliths can also be removed using electrohydraulic, ultrasonographic, or continuous wave or pulsed dye laser lithotripsy [38–40]. Pulsed dye laser lithotripsy can be performed transendoscopically with the horse standing. An ischial urethrot-omy, however, may be required to remove fragments.

Because almost all uroliths of horses are composed of calcium carbonate [32], a low-calcium diet is recommended to prevent recurrence. The diet should meet but not exceed the horse's calcium requirements [41]. This can be accomplished by feeding mature grass pasture or hay or a cereal-grain hay and grain with no added calcium [41]. Early growth grass and legume forages should be avoided. Other recommendations for preventing recurrence of urolithiasis usually involve supplementing feed with urinary acidifiers or salt. Urinary acidification with ammonium chloride, ammo-nium sulfate, or ascorbic acid is often prescribed to prevent recurrence of urinary tract calculi [35,42]. These urinary acidifiers are unpalatable to most horses, however, and there are no studies that compare the likelihood of recurrence of calculi between horses that have received urinary acidifiers and horses that have not received urinary acidifiers. The urinary pH at which formation of calcium carbonate calculi is inhibited in the horse is not known. Urinary acidifiers decrease the dietary cation-anion balance, which is claimed to increases the horse's calcium urinary excretion; thus, they may be more harmful than beneficial [41]. In one study, however, horses fed a diet with a low calcium/phosphorus ratio and a low dietary cation-anion balance did not develop hypercalciuria [43]. A more practical approach to prevent recurrence of urolithiasis may be to promote increased consumption of water and urine output by increasing the salt content of the ration. Diuresis in horses can be promoted by adding salt to the daily ration, but there is little information to indicate the amount of salt that must be in the ration to increase water consumption and urine output. Addition of 200 to 500 g of salt to the diet was recommended to increase water consumption and urine output in horses (1.7%–4.4% salt in the ration of a 450-kg horse consuming 2.5% of its body weight) [44]. In a metabolism study, however, horses consuming a diet containing 5% salt showed no greater water consumption or urine output compared with horses that consumed a diet containing 1% salt [45]. Sheep fed rations of 4% or greater concentrations of salt had a significantly lower incidence of urolithiasis than did sheep fed a urinary alkalizing ration [46]. Sheep fed the high-salt diets had a significant increase in urine output, but the decreased incidence of urolithiasis was also speculated to be caused by a direct effect of salt on inhibition of formation of uroliths.

Several long-term follow-up evaluations of horses that had calculi removed by celiocystotomy indicate that recurrence of cystic urolithiasis is not likely [36,47]; however, in one retrospective study, 12 (41%) of 29 horses had recurrence of urolithiasis within 1 to 32 months [32]. Recurrence of a cystic urolith may be more likely if the urolith was fragmented before removal [32,48]. If a cystic urolith is fragmented for removal, the bladder should be re-examined by endoscopy after surgery to ensure that no fragments of the calculus are left to act as a nidus for formation of new cystic uroliths.

In a recent report [49], four horses and a burro with recurrent urolithiasis were found to have unilateral pyelonephritis. Because recurrence of urolithiasis of these animals was suspected to be the consequence of disease of the upper portion of the urinary tract, the recommendation was made that horses presented for urolithiasis should be examined for disease of the upper urinary tract. At a minimum, the examination should consist of renal ultrasonography, endoscopy of the urethra and bladder, and submission of urine for culture.

Pyelonephritis

Pyelonephritis, which is a suppurative bacterial infection of the renal pelvis and parenchyma, was thought to be the cause of severe hematuria for seven horses with unilateral or bilateral renal hemorrhage [50]. The horses in that report, however, had none of the typical clinical signs (azotemia, polydipsia and polyuria, leukocytosis, and fever) or predisposing causes (urethral trauma, sorghum cystitis, uroliths, or other causes of obstruction of the flow of urine) of pyelonephritis [27]. A renal biopsy of one of these horses supported an ultrasonographic diagnosis of pyelonephritis; however, for the other horses, the diagnosis was based primarily on ultrasonographic images typical of pyelonephritis in other species [51]. Because the diagnosis was unsupported by urinalysis or culture for many of these horses, the conclusions of this report are controversial. Urinary tract infection, however, may exist in the absence of pyuria [7], and it has been speculated that pyelonephritis may be underdiagnosed as a cause of renal disease in the horse [52].

Characteristic changes seen during ultrasonography of equine pyelonephritis include increased renal echogenicity, abnormal renal outline, loss of corticomedullary distinction, detection of a large amount of echogenic to hyperechoic debris in the renal pelvis, and pyelectasia (dilatation of the renal pelvis) [52,53]. Because only a few ultrasonographic changes associated with pyelonephritis of horses are likely to be present at any given time, ultrasonographic evidence of pyelonephritis may increase if the kidneys are sequentially examined ultrasonographically [50]. Biopsy of a kidney with an abnormal ultrasonographic appearance would likely aid in the diagnosis of pyelonephritis.

Trimethoprim-sulfonamide, or penicillin, is probably an appropriate antimicrobial drug for treatment for horses with pyelonephritis, but bacterial culture of urine and antimicrobial sensitivity testing of cultured bacteria are indicated. Horses with hematuria caused by renal leptospiral infection may respond to treatment with penicillin [54]. The recommended minimum duration of antimicrobial therapy for horses with infection of the upper portion of the urinary tract is 3 weeks [55]. Intravenously administered electrolyte solution and repeated blood transfusions may be necessary for some horses with severe urinary blood loss. In a retrospective study of seven horses with pyelonephritis and macroscopic hematuria, all horses had recurrence of hematuria (John Schumacher, unpublished data, 2002) [50].

Idiopathic hematuria

A syndrome of idiopathic hematuria that primarily affects Arabian horses has been described (Dr. Harold Schott, personal communication, February 12, 2007) [21,56] that closely resembled the clinical findings of horses with hematuria suspected to be caused by pyelonephritis (most of which were also Arabian) [50]. Horses with idiopathic hematuria had severe renal hemorrhage that was usually unilateral but was occasionally bilateral, with no other signs of disease. The diagnosis was made by exclusion of known causes of renal hemorrhage; in five horses diagnosed with this condition, there was no evidence of upper urinary tract infection, even during histologic examination of some affected kidneys. Treatment of horses with idiopathic hematuria may be warranted because some have remission of clinical signs. Suggested treatment is supportive care that may involve blood transfusion. When the condition appears to be unilateral, nephrectomy may be indicated. Three Arabian horses, however, developed renal hemorrhage in the remaining kidney after undergoing nephrectomy (Dr. Harold Schott, personal communication, February 12, 2007) [21]. Arabian horses undergoing unilateral nephrectomy to treat this condition may have a poor prognosis for recovery.

Verminous nephritis

Hematuria in horses caused by renal infection with *Halicephalobus gingivalis* [57–60] or *Strongylus vulgaris* [61] has been reported. *H gingivalis*, previously known as *Micronema deletrix* and synonymous with *H deletrix* [62], is a saprophytic nematode that rarely causes disease in horses. The nematode can invade the central nervous system to cause neurologic signs; bone to cause osteomyelitis; and the kidneys, wherein it creates granulomas that may cause hematuria. The nematode may be found during urinalysis of affected horses [63] or during histologic examination of renal tissue obtained by biopsy [64]. Horses with renal disease caused by *H gingivalis* often have signs of neurologic disease or osteomyelitis.

The ultrasonographic appearance of renal granulomas caused by *H gingivalis* has been described as similar in echogenicity to the renal cortex [52,65]. One kidney, however, had a normal appearance during ultrasonographic examination but contained firm renal masses when examined during necropsy [52]; for another kidney, the ultrasonographic image of a granuloma containing *H gingivalis* appeared anechoic to hypoechoic relative to the renal cortex [65].

Horses suspected to have a renal infection of *H gingivalis* should be treated with an anthelmintic that has larvicidal activity. Inflammation associated with death of the nematode may cause clinical signs of renal infection soon after administration of an anthelmintic [60,66]. Consequently, horses thought to be infected with *H gingivalis* should be treated with an anti-inflammatory drug, in addition to an anthelmintic with larvicidal activity. Although no successful treatment of horses with verminous nephritis has been reported [60,65,67], similar treatment of horses with verminous encephalitis is often successful [63]. Unilateral nephrectomy resolved clinical signs in a donkey with a renal infection caused by *H gingivalis* [65].

Renal and vesicular neoplasia

Neoplastic invasion of the renal vasculature is an uncommon cause of hematuria of horses [68]. Adenocarcinoma (also known as a renal cell carcinoma) and lymphosarcoma are the most common tumors affecting the kidney, but adenocarcinoma is more likely than lymphosarcoma to cause hematuria [52]. An antemortem diagnosis of renal neoplasia is unlikely if ultrasonographic examination of the neoplastic kidney is not possible, unless the left kidney is affected and has a change in its palpable characteristics [69]. Large masses of mixed echogenicity are typical of adenocarcinomas [52,69]. Renal adenocarcinomas in horses are usually inoperable because the neoplasm is often not diagnosed until the tumor has metastasized to the liver, lungs, and adjacent lymph nodes [27].

Squamous cell and transitional cell carcinomas are reported to cause hematuria in horses [70–72]. Clinical findings of horses with bladder tumors are similar to those of horses with cystic calculi (ie, hematuria and stranguria with a palpable mass in the bladder). Bladder tumors are readily diagnosed by identifying neoplastic cells during urinalysis or by endoscopic examination of the bladder. Tissue samples for cytologic or histologic examination can be obtained using the biopsy instrument of the endoscope [70]. The prognosis for survival of horses with neoplasia of the bladder is poor; however, in one case, intravesical administration of 5-fluorouracil arrested the growth of squamous cell carcinoma [70]. Intravesical therapy using chemotherapeutic agents, such as methotrexate, vinblastine, doxorubicin, and cisplatin, which are used to treat people with bladder cancer [73], has not been reported for the horse.

Blister beetle (cantharidin) toxicosis

Hematuria is not a common clinical finding in horses with blister beetle toxicosis [74], but this condition should be considered as a cause of hematuria for horses fed alfalfa hay that have concurrent signs of abdominal pain. Hematuria caused by ingestion of blister beetles occurs late in the syndrome [75]; by that time, other clinical signs usually make the cause of hematuria obvious. The author is aware, however, of a horse with cantharidin toxicosis that had macroscopic hematuria for several days with subtle signs of abdominal pain (sweating and rapid pulse and respiration) (Dr. Fred Caldwell, personal communication, January 12, 2007). Clinical signs depend on the amount of cantharidin ingested and range from signs of severe abdominal pain and shock to mild colic and depression. Cantharidin, the toxic principle of blister beetles, is irritating to the digestive and urinary tracts. Irritation of the urinary tract may cause pollakiuria and hemorrhage of the urinary mucosa [76]. Typical and significant clinicopathologic findings in horses with blister beetle toxicosis are increased serum CK activity and decreased serum concentrations of calcium and magnesium. The finding of a low concentration of serum calcium in any horse with colic should arouse suspicion of blister beetle toxicosis.

Poisoning by ingestion of the dead beetle occurs almost exclusively in horses fed alfalfa hay, but horses fed other types of hay contaminated with weeds used by the beetle as a food source (eg, nightshade plants) may also develop blister beetle toxicosis [77]. Beetles (Fig. 8) are not always found during a search of the contaminated hay; thus, the condition is definitively diagnosed by finding cantharidin in the urine, stomach contents, or contaminated hay using high-pressure liquid chromatography, gas chromatography, or mass spectrometry [77,78]. To detect cantharidin, at least 500 mL of urine or 200 g of stomach contents should be submitted to a toxicology laboratory in a refrigerated container. Samples should be collected early in the course of the condition before concentrations of cantharidin decrease

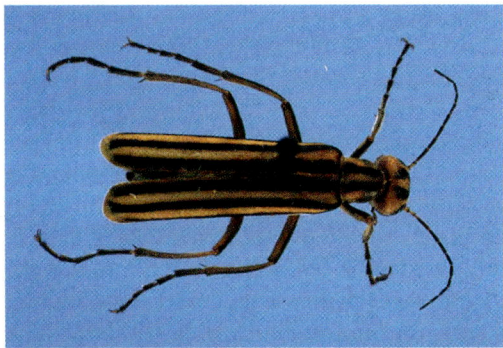

Fig. 8. Blister beetles range from 0.74 to 2 cm in length and are often black, striped, or spotted.

to negligible levels [76]. Because litigation often follows a diagnosis of blister beetle toxicosis, the condition should be definitively diagnosed.

Treatment of horses with blister beetle toxicosis includes repeated administration of mineral oil by nasogastric tube because cantharidin is lipid soluble. Diuresis of affected horses with intravenously administered balanced polyionic fluids (with calcium added if the horse is hypocalcemic) and furosemide may be beneficial because cantharidin is excreted by way of the kidneys.

Less common causes of macroscopic hematuria

Grossly evident hematuria was reported in three neonatal foals that had developed a hematoma within the bladder and urachus [79]. Affected foals had stranguria that was likely the result of urinary tract obstruction. Trauma to the umbilicus during the periparturient period with damage to the vessels within that structure resulted in retrograde bleeding into the bladder. During abdominal ultrasonography of these foals, a homogeneous or heterogeneous echogenic mass was seen within the lumen of the bladder and the urachus was enlarged with a heterogenic echo pattern. One foal was successfully treated medically with intravenously administered fluids to promote diuresis. Other foals were treated surgically by removing the cystic hematoma, along with the umbilical remnants and bladder apex. Differential diagnoses listed by the authors of that report included urinary tract obstruction or rupture, drug toxicosis, acute renal tubular necrosis, sepsis, congenital malformations, and leptospirosis.

Macroscopic hematuria was reported in horses with anuric or oliguric renal failure that also had intravascular hemolysis [80,81]. Histologic lesions found during necropsy included arteriolar microangiopathy. These cases were compared with the hemolytic-uremic syndrome of human beings, a syndrome of renal failure and hematuria caused by verotoxins produced by specific types of *Escherichia coli* and associated with the consumption of raw milk or undercooked hamburger [82]. For horses with this syndrome, bacterial toxins, or possibly other agents, may have caused endothelial damage in glomerular capillary loops and small arterioles, leading to renal failure and hemorrhage. Intravascular hemolysis was likely caused by damage to red blood cells as they flowed through fibrin strands deposited in small renal vessels.

This syndrome should be suspected in horses that have hematuria, intravascular hemolysis with red blood cell fragmentation, and clinicopathologic evidence of renal failure. Although horses reported to have hemolytic uremic-like syndrome died, treatment of affected horses should include intravenously administered polyionic fluids and diuretics to induce polyuria. Urine discolored pink from renal hemorrhage and hemoglobinuria has been observed in horses with purpura hemorrhagica (Dr. Harold Schott, personal communication, February 12, 2007). In these horses, it is likely that a similar syndrome of hemorrhage and red blood cell fragmentation occurred in kidneys affected with glomerulonephritis.

Macroscopic hematuria in horses can be caused by chronic administration of NSAIDs, usually phenylbutazone, to dehydrated or hypotensive horses or when it is administered in excess of recommended doses [16,83,84]. Combination therapy using NSAIDS, such as phenylbutazone and flunixin meglumine, may potentiate the detrimental effects of these drugs [85]. Chronic or excessive administration of NSAIDs causes decreased renal medullary blood flow, which can result in medullary and pelvic necrosis. Increased echogenicity of the renal papilla and echogenic debris in the renal pelvis may be seen on ultrasonography of affected kidneys [52]. The diagnosis is supported by clinicopathologic evidence of renal failure and a history of administration of NSAIDs. Treatment of affected horses involves discontinuation of administration of NSAIDs and correction of fluid volume and electrolyte deficits.

Vascular anomalies that can be congenital or acquired are a rare cause of hematuria in the horse. A congenital renal arteriovenous fistula was a cause of hematuria in a foal [86]. The hematuria and renal lesion in this foal resolved within weeks, but another horse with a renal vascular anomaly did not develop hematuria until it was mature [87]. A fistula between an aneurysm of the terminal aorta and a ureter was the cause of hematuria in another foal [88]. The cause of the vascular anomaly in this foal was not determined.

Diagnosis of vascular anomalies is aided by ultrasonographic examination of the urinary tract. Color-flow Doppler ultrasonography may be particularly useful in diagnosis of vascular anomalies [89]. If the contralateral kidney is functioning normally, the kidney responsible for the hematuria can be removed [87], but more conservative treatment may be effective [89]. Creating a thrombus within the vascular lesion by selective renal arterial embolization (a procedure during which an occlusion device is placed, using fluoroscopic guidance, within the vascular lesion) may be effective in resolving hematuria. Spontaneous formation of a thrombus within a renal vascular anomaly resulted in resolution of hematuria in a foal [86].

Macroscopic hematuria is observed occasionally in exercising horses. Repeated concussion of the bladder during exercise can be sufficient to cause mucosal damage and hemorrhage. A small amount of urine in the bladder may act as a cushion to prevent this injury; therefore, urination immediately before exercise may predispose to injury of the bladder mucosa [89].

Myoglobinuria

Myoglobinuria is the result of muscle necrosis caused by trauma; immune-mediated myopathy; exertional rhabdomyolysis; polysaccharide storage myopathy; toxic drugs, such as monensin; toxic plants, such as coffee senna and white snake root; and idiopathic causes, such as atypical myopathy. Acute renal failure is a complication of myoglobinuria. Mechanisms of myoglobin-induced nephrotoxicity include direct toxicity of the proximal tubular epithelium caused by free chelatable iron and obstruction of the distal tubules with precipitates of myoglobin [90,91]. Because myoglobin chelates nitric oxide, it also has a vasoconstrictive effect to cause renal ischemia [91]. Prevention and treatment of myoglobinuric renal failure involve maintenance of circulating blood volume by adequate fluid replacement. Furosemide is administered to promote diuresis and enhance elimination of pigment. In people, alkalinization of the urine by means of addition of sodium bicarbonate to the intravenous fluids has been suggested because acidic urine favors myoglobin nephrotoxicity [91]. Because equine urine is normally alkaline, similar treatment of affected horses is probably not necessary.

Hemoglobinuria

Hemoglobinuria is the result of intravascular hemolysis caused by infectious disease involving the hemopoietic system, ingestion of compounds toxic to red blood cells, and immune-mediated diseases [92]. Infectious diseases that cause hemoglobinuria in the horse include equine piroplasmosis, equine infectious anemia, and equine ehrlichiosis. The most common toxic cause is ingestion of wilted red maple leaves. Immune-mediated hemolysis and hemoglobinuria can be idiopathic or caused by bacterial infections, drugs, neoplasia, and colostral-derived antibodies to red blood cells (neonatal isoerythrolysis).

Acute renal failure is a complication of hemoglobinuria, and the mechanisms of hemoglobin-induced nephrotoxicity are the same as those causing myoglobin-induced nephrotoxicity (see section on myoglobinuria) [90,91].

References

[1] Valberg SJ. Diagnostic approach to muscle disorders. Proceedings of the American Association of Equine Practitioners 2006;52:340–6.

[2] Duncan RJ, Prasse KW. Urinary system. In: Veterinary laboratory medicine. 2nd edition. Ames (IA): The Iowa State University Press; 1986. p. 153–73.

[3] Coffman JR. Urinalysis. In: Equine clinical chemistry and pathophysiology. Bonner Springs (KS): Veterinary Medicine Publishing Company; 1981. p. 180–7.

[4] Wright B. Horse news and views—August 2003. Available at: www.omafra.gov.on.ca/english/livestock/horses/news/aug03. Accessed December 29, 2006.

[5] Neizen JH, Barry TN, Wilson PR, et al. Red urine from red deer grazed on pure red clover swards. N Z Vet J 1992;40(4):164–7.

[6] Anon. Orange-red urine seen in dairy cows. Surveillance 1983;10(2):6.

[7] Kohn CW, Chew DJ. Laboratory diagnosis and characterization of renal disease in horses. Vet Clin North Am Equine Pract 1987;3(3):585–615.

[8] Kohn CW, Strasser SL. 24-Hour renal clearance and excretion of endogenous substances in the mare. Am J Vet Res 1986;47(6):1332–7.

[9] Traub-Dargatz JL, McKinnon AO. Adjunct methods of examination of the urogenital tract. Vet Clin North Am Equine Pract 1988;4(3):339–58.

[10] Schott HC, Hodgson DR, Bayly WM. Ureteral catheterization in the horse. Equine Veterinary Education 1990;2:140–3.

[11] Rantanen NW. Diseases of the kidney. Vet Clin North Am Equine Pract 1986;2(1):89–103.

[12] Bayly WM, Pardis MR, Reed SM. Equine renal biopsy: indications, technique, interpretation and complications. Mod Vet Pract 1980;61:763–8.

[13] Barratt-Boyes SM, Spensley MS, Nyland TG, et al. Ultrasound localization and guidance for renal biopsy in the horse. Veterinary Radiology 1991;32(3):121–6.

[14] Lloyd KC, Wheat JD, Ryan AM, et al. Ulceration in the proximal portion of the urethra as a cause of hematuria of horses: four cases 1978–1985. J Am Vet Med Assoc 1989;194(9):1324–6.

[15] Schumacher J, Varner DD, Schmitz DG, et al. Urethral defects in geldings with hematuria and stallions with hemospermia. Vet Surg 1995;24(3):250–4.

[16] Divers TJ. Equine renal system. In: Smith BP, editor. Large animal internal medicine. 2nd edition. Philadelphia: CV Mosby; 1996. p. 953–74.

[17] Sisson S, Grossman JD. The male urethra. In: The anatomy of domestic animals. 4th edition. Philadelphia: WB Saunders; 1953. p. 594–6.

[18] Taintor JS, Schumacher J, Schumacher J, et al. Comparison of pressure within the corpus spongiosum penis during urination between stallions and geldings. Equine Vet J 2004; 6(4):362–4.

[19] Schott HC. Hematuria. In: Reed SM, Bayly WM, editors. Equine internal medicine. Philadelphia: WB Saunders; 1998. p. 890–5.

[20] Sullins KE, Bertone JJ, Voss JL, et al. Treatment of hemospermia in stallions: a discussion of 18 cases. Compendium of Continuing Education for the Practicing Veterinarian 1988;10(12):1396–403.

[21] Schott HC. Urinary tract infections. In: Reed SM, Bayly WM, editors. Equine internal medicine. Philadelphia: WB Saunders; 1998. p. 875–80.

[22] Schott HC, Varner DD. Urinary tract. In: Traub-Dargatz JL, Brown CM, editors. Equine endoscopy. 2nd edition. St. Louis (MO): Mosby-Year Book, Inc.; 1997. p. 187–203.

[23] Schumacher J, Schumacher J, Schmitz D. Macroscopic hematuria of horses. Equine Veterinary Education 2002;14(4):201–10.

[24] Bridges ER. The use of ivermectin to treat genital cutaneous habronemiasis in a stallion. Compendium of Continuing Education for the Practicing Veterinarian 1985;7:S94–7.

[25] Herd RP, Donaham JC. Efficacy of ivermectin against cutaneous Draschia and Habronema infection (summer sores) in horses. Am J Vet Res 1981;42:1952–5.

[26] Stick JA. Amputation of the equine urethral process affected with habronemiasis. Vet Med Small Anim Clin 1979;74:1453–7.

[27] Rooney JR, Robertson JL. Urinary tract. In: Equine pathology. Ames (IA): Iowa State University Press; 1996. p. 285–6.

[28] Divers TJ. Commentary, clinical case conference. J Am Vet Med Assoc 1995;207(4):420.

[29] Byars TD, Simpson JS, Divers TJ, et al. Percutaneous nephrostomy in short-term management of ureterolithiasis and renal dysfunction in a filly. J Am Vet Med Assoc 1989;195(4):499–501.

[30] Hope WD, Wilson JH, Hager DA, et al. Chronic renal failure associated with bilateral nephroliths and ureteroliths in a two-year-old Thoroughbred colt. Equine Vet J 1989;21(3):228–31.

[31] Ehnen SJ, Divers TJ, Gillette D, et al. Obstructive nephrolithiasis and ureterolithiasis associated with chronic renal failure in horses: eight cases (1981-1987). J Am Vet Med Assoc 1990;197(2):249–53.

[32] Laverty S, Pascoe JR, Ling GV, et al. Urolithiasis in 68 horses. Vet Surg 1992;21(1):56–62.

[33] Divers TJ, Yeager AE. The value of ultrasonographic examination in the diagnosis and management of renal diseases in horses. Equine Veterinary Education 1995;7(6):334–41.

[34] Frank ER. Vesicular calculi in the equine. In: Veterinary surgery. 7th edition. Minneapolis (MN): Burgess Publishing Co.; 1964. p. 308–10.

[35] DeBowes RM, Nyrop KA, Boulton CH. Cystic calculi in the horse. Compendium of Continuing Education for the Practicing Veterinarian 1984;6:S268–73.

[36] Holt PE, Pearson H. Urolithiasis in the horse—a review of 13 cases. Equine Vet J 1984;16:31–4.

[37] Hackett RP, Vaughan JT, Tennant BC. The urinary system. In: Mansmann RA, McAllister ES, Pratt PW, editors. Equine medicine and surgery, vol. 2. 3rd editionSanta Barbara (CA): American Veterinary Publications; 1985. p. 907–22.

[38] Eustace RA, Hunt JM, Brearley MJ. Electrohydraulic lithotripsy for the treatment of cystic calculus in two geldings. Equine Vet J 1988;20(3):221–3.

[39] Rodger LD, Carlson GP, Moran ME, et al. Resolution of a left ureteral stone using electrohydraulic lithotripsy in a thoroughbred colt. J Vet Intern Med 1995;9(4):280–2.

[40] Howard RD, Pleasant RS, May KA. Pulsed dye laser lithotripsy for treatment of urolithiasis in two geldings. J Am Vet Med Assoc 1998;212(10):1600–3.

[41] Lewis LD. Sick horse feeding and nutritional support. In: Equine clinical nutrition: feeding and care. Philadelphia: Williams & Wilkins; 1995. p. 389–419.

[42] Wood T, Weckman PA, Henry PA, et al. Equine urine pH: normal population distributions and methods of acidification. Equine Vet J 1990;22(2):118–21, 42.

[43] McKenzie EC, Valberg SJ, Godden SM, et al. Plasma and urine electrolyte and mineral concentrations in Thoroughbred horses with recurrent exertional rhabdomyolysis after consumption of diets varying in cation-anion balance. Am J Vet Res 2002;63(7):1053–60.

[44] Keller H. Diseases of the urinary system. In: Wintzer HJ, editor. Equine diseases. New York: Springer Verlag; 1986. p. 148–59.

[45] Schryver HF, Parker MT, Daniluk PD, et al. Salt consumption and the effects of salt on mineral metabolism in horses. Cornell Vet 1987;77:122–31.

[46] Udall RH. Studies on urolithiasis. V. The effects of urinary pH and dietary sodium chloride on the urinary excretion of proteins and the incidence of calculosis. Am J Vet Res 1962;23:1241–5.

[47] Lowe JE. Long term results of cystotomy for removal of uroliths from horses. J Am Vet Med Assoc 1965;147(3):147.

[48] Lowe JE. Surgical removal of equine uroliths via the laparoscopy approach. J Am Vet Med Assoc 1961;139(3):345–8.

[49] Schott HC. Recurrent urolithiasis associated with unilateral pyelonephritis in 5 equids. Proceedings of the American Association of Equine Practitioners 2002;48:136–7.

[50] Kisthardt KK, Schumacher J, Finn-Bodner ST, et al. Severe renal hemorrhage caused by pyelonephritis in 7 horses: clinical and ultrasonographic evaluation. Can Vet J 1999;40:571–6.

[51] Biller DS, Schenkman DI, Bortnowski H. Ultrasonographic appearance of renal infarcts in a dog. J Am Anim Hosp Assoc 1991;27:370–2.

[52] Reef VB. Abnormalities of the kidneys. In: Equine diagnostic ultrasound. Philadelphia: WB Saunders; 1998. p. 291–304.

[53] Mathews HK, Joal RL. A review of equine imaging techniques. Vet Radiol Ultrasound 1996; 37(3):163–73.

[54] Bernard WV, Williams D, Tuttle PA, et al. Hematuria and leptospiruria in a foal. J Am Vet Med Assoc 1993;203(2):276–8.

[55] Prescott JF, Baggot JD. Special considerations. In: Prescott JF, Baggot JD, editors. Antimicrobial therapy in veterinary medicine. Ames (IA): Iowa State University Press; 1993. p. 334–91.

[56] Schott HC, Hines MT. Severe urinary tract hemorrhage in two horses [letters to the editor]. J Am Vet Med Assoc 1994;204(9):1320.

[57] Rubin HL, Woodard JC. Equine infection with Micronema deletrix. J Am Vet Med Assoc 1974;165(3):256–8.

[58] Keg PR, Mirck MH, Dik KJ, et al. Micronema deletrix infection in a Shetland pony stallion. Equine Vet J 1984;16:471–5.

[59] Blunden AS, Khalil LF, Webbon PM. Halicephalobus deletrix infection in a horse. Equine Vet J 1987;19:255–60.

[60] Ruggles AJ, Beech J, Gillette DM, et al. Disseminated Halicephalobus deletrix infection in a horse. J Am Vet Med Assoc 1993;203(4):550–2.

[61] Mahaffey LW, Adam NM. Strongylus vulgaris in the urinary tract of a foal and some observations upon the habits of the parasite. Veterinary Record 1975;22:716–7.

[62] Anderson RC, Linder KE, Peregrine AS. Halicephalobus gingivalis (Stephanski 1954) from a fatal infection in a horse in Ontario, Canada with comments on the validity of H. deletrix and a review of the genus. Parasite 1998;5:255–61.

[63] Mayhew IG. Verminous encephalitis. In: Large animal neurology, a handbook for veterinary clinicians. Philadelphia: Lea & Febiger; 1989. p. 92–3.

[64] Kinde H, Mathews M, Ash L, et al. Halicephalobus gingivalis (H. deletrix) infection in two horses in southern California. J Vet Diagn Invest 2000;12(2):162–5.

[65] Schmitz DG, Chaffin MK. What is your diagnosis? J Am Vet Med Assoc 2004;225(11): 1667–8.

[66] Alstad AD, Berg JE, Samuel C. Disseminated Micronema deletrix infection in the horse. J Am Vet Med Assoc 1979;174(3):264–6.

[67] Trostle SS, Wilson DG, Steinberg H, et al. Antemortem diagnosis and attempted treatment of (Halicephalobus) Micronema deletrix infection in a horse. Can Vet J 1993;34:117–8.

[68] Brown PJ, Holt PE. Primary renal cell carcinoma in four horses. Equine Vet J 1985;17(6): 473–7.

[69] Ramirez S, Seahorn TL. Ultrasonography as an aid in the diagnosis of renal cell carcinoma in a horse. Vet Radiol Ultrasound 1996;37(5):383–6.

[70] Fischer AT, Spier S, Carlson GP, et al. Neoplasia of the equine bladder as a cause of hematuria. J Am Vet Med Assoc 1985;186(12):1294–6.

[71] Turner RM, Love CC, McDonnell SM, et al. Use of imipramine hydrochloride for treatment of urospermia in a stallion with a dysfunctional bladder. J Am Vet Med Assoc 1995;207(12): 1602–6.

[72] Patterson-Kane JC, Tramontin RR, Giles RC, et al. Transitional cell carcinoma of the urinary bladder in a Thoroughbred, with abdominal dissemination. Vet Pathol 2000;37:692–5.

[73] Presti JC, Stoller ML, Carroll PR. Urology. In: Tierney LM, McPhee SJ, Papadakis MA, editors. Current medical diagnosis and treatment. 37th edition. Samford (CT): Appleton & Lange; 1998. p. 878–915.

[74] Helman RG, Edwards WC. Clinical features of blister beetle poisoning in equids: 70 cases (1983–1986). J Am Vet Med Assoc 1997;211(8):1018–21.

[75] Panciera RJ. Cantharidin (blister beetle) poisoning. In: Mansmann RA, McAllister ES, editors. Equine medicine and surgery. 3rd edition. Santa Barbara (CA): American Veterinary Publications; 1982. p. 203–4.

[76] Schmitz DG, Reagor JC. Cantharidine (blister beetle) toxicosis. In: Robinson NE, editor. Current therapy in equine medicine. 2nd edition. Philadelphia: WB Saunders; 1987. p. 120–2.

[77] Ray AC, Kyle ALG, Murphy MJ, et al. Etiologic agents, incidence, and improved diagnostic methods of cantharidin toxicosis in horses. Am J Vet Res 1989;50(2):187–91.

[78] Osweiler GD. Zootoxins. In: Toxicology. Philadelphia: Williams and Wilkins; 1996. p. 437–44.

[79] Arnold CE, Chaffin MK, Rush BR. Hematuria associated with cystic hematomas in three neonatal foals. J Am Vet Med Assoc 2005;227(5):778–80.

[80] MacLachlan NJ, Divers TJ. Hemolytic anemia and fibroid changes of renal vessels in a horse. J Am Vet Med Assoc 1982;181(7):1716–7.

[81] Morris CF, Robertson JL, Mann PC, et al. Hemolytic uremic-like syndrome in two horses. J Am Vet Med Assoc 1987;191(11):1453–4.

[82] Martin ML, Shipman LD. More on hemolytic uremic-like syndrome [letters to the editor]. J Am Vet Med Assoc 1988;192(11):1493.

[83] Behm RJ, Berg IE. Hematuria caused by renal medullary necrosis in a horse. Compendium of Continuing Education for the Practicing Veterinarian 1987;9(6):698–703.

[84] Edwards JF, Carter GK. Severe renal pelvic necrosis and hematuria of Arabian horses associated with possible analgesic nephrosis. Proceedings of the 42nd Annual Meeting of the American College of Veterinary Pathologists 1991:45.

[85] Reed SK, Messer NT, Tessman RK, et al. Effects of phenylbutazone alone or in combination with flunixin meglumine on blood protein concentrations in horses. Am J Vet Res 2006;67(3):398–402.

[86] Schott HC, Barbee DD, Hines MT, et al. Renal arteriovenous malformation in a quarter horse foal. J Vet Intern Med 1996;10(4):204–6.

[87] Divers TJ. Congenital and familial diseases of the kidney. In: Colahan PT, Merritt AM, Mayhew IG, editors. Equine medicine and surgery. 5th edition. St. Louis (MO): Mosby; 1999. p. 1769–70.

[88] Latimer FG, Magnus R, Duncan RB. Arterioureteral fistula in a colt. Equine Vet J 1991; 23(6):483–4.

[89] Schott HC, Hodgson DR, Bayly WM. Haematuria, pigmenturia and proteinuria in exercising horses. Equine Vet J 1995;27(1):67–72.

[90] Humphreys MH. Pigment and crystal-induced acute renal failure. In: Jacobson HR, Striker G, Klahr S, editors. The principles and practice of nephrology. St. Louis (MO): BC Decker Inc.; 1991. p. 650.

[91] Zager RA. Rhabdomyolysis and myohemoglobinuric acute renal failure. Kidney Int 1996; 49:314–26.

[92] Morris DD. Review of anemia in horses, part II: pathophysiologic mechanisms, specific diseases and treatment. Equine Practice 1989;2(5):34–46.

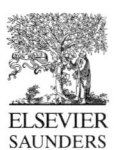

VETERINARY
CLINICS
Equine Practice

ELSEVIER
SAUNDERS

Vet Clin Equine 23 (2007) 677–690

Toxins Affecting the Urinary System

David G. Schmitz, DVM, MS

*Department of Veterinary Large Animal Clinical Sciences, College of Veterinary Medicine,
Texas A&M University, College Station, TX 77843–4475, USA*

Plants

Sorghum

An ataxia-cystitis syndrome in horses has been associated with the ingestion of *Sorghum* species and certain hybrid Sudan grasses [1,2]. Horses grazing the plant can be affected, and toxicity is more likely to occur when the plant is young and rapidly growing, but second-growth and mature plants can also cause toxicity. Signs of toxicity may develop after a grazing period of 1 week to several months, and the occurrence of toxicity may increase during periods of medium to high rainfall. No cases of toxicity have been recognized when grazing the plant after the date of the first frost, and feeding well-cured *Sorghum* species hay has not resulted in signs of toxicity [3].

The primary clinical signs are those of posterior ataxia and urinary incontinence, often associated with cystitis. Urinary incontinence characterized by continual urine dribbling is prominent in both genders, and scalding of the dependent skin is common. The urinary bladder is usually distended and atonic, resulting in moderate to severe cystitis. Inflammation of the urethra and ureters may also develop, and ascending pyelonephritis usually contributes to the cause of death in horses that die from the condition [3].

The clinical signs are a result of axonal degeneration and demyelination of nerve fibers in the spinal cord, especially in the lumbar and sacral segments. The substance in *Sorghum* species responsible for this neuronal change is unknown, but sublethal amounts of hydrogen cyanide have been suggested as being causative [1]. Cystitis usually develops secondarily as an ascending infection because of urinary retention and failure of the bladder to contract and void urine.

Diagnosis of the condition is usually based on appropriate clinical signs, a history of grazing the plant, and exclusion of other causes of similar

E-mail address: dschmitz@cvm.tamu.edu

doi:10.1016/j.cveq.2007.09.001   *vetequine.theclinics.com* clinical signs. No definitive diagnostic test is available, and treatment is supportive and symptomatic [3]. Horses should be immediately removed from grazing the plant. Appropriate antibiotic treatment for bacterial urinary tract infections should be instituted, and urinary scald dermatitis can be topically treated. Urinary bladder catheterization or frequent manual decompression of the bladder may also aid in resolution of the cystitis.

Affected horses usually show gradual improvement in clinical signs over several weeks to months once they are removed from grazing the plant, but complete recovery may not occur.

Oxalate toxicosis

Plants, particularly those of the Chenopodiaceae family, are the most common source of oxalates for horses. These plants are generally unpalatable to horses, however, so plant-associated oxalate intoxication is rare. These plants contain varied amounts of soluble oxalates, usually in the form of potassium or sodium salts, but the following plants contain large amounts of soluble oxalates:

Amaranthus: spp pigweed
Halogeton glomeratus: halogeton
Sarcobatus vermiculatus: black greasewood
Rumex spp: sorrel, dock
Salsola kali: Russian thistle
Beta vulgaris: beet, mangold
Chenopodium album: lambsquarters
Oxalis spp: wood sorrel, soursob
Portulaca oleracea: purslane
Rheum rhaponticum: rhubarb

Sarcobatus and *Halogeton* seem to be the primary offenders in range animals in the western United States [4].

The incidence of toxicosis may be highest in the fall and winter months, because oxalates accumulate in the plants throughout the growing season [5]. Leaves contain the highest content of oxalates, with a lesser amount found in seeds, and minimal amounts present in stems. The nonfatal toxic dose of sodium oxalate for adult horses is approximately 200 g/d for 8 days [4].

Renal toxicity occurs with chronic ingestion of oxalates. Oxalates combine with serum calcium ions to form insoluble calcium oxalate. These insoluble crystals can lodge in renal tubules, producing tubular blockage and necrosis [4].

Definitive diagnosis may be difficult, but urinalysis may reveal the presence of characteristic calcium oxalate crystals on microscopic examination. Treatment is usually of little value after clinical signs have appeared. Symptomatic therapy, including balanced electrolyte solutions, can be initiated to aid diuresis, and diuretics may be beneficial in the volume-loaded patient. Prevention is primarily aimed at limiting access to the plants by means of providing adequate suitable sources of feed [4].

Oak

Oak (*Quercus* spp) poisoning is reportedly rare in horses [6]. Toxicity can occur when large quantities of the flowers, leaf buds, or acorns are ingested. These parts of the plant have higher concentrations of tannic and gallic acids, which are toxic to renal tubular epithelial cells. Clinical signs are not limited to the urinary system, and include depression, acute onset of abdominal pain, straining and bloody diarrhea, hematuria, and increased heart and respiratory rates. The major clinicopathologic abnormalities noted are dehydration, azotemia, hyperphosphatemia, hypoproteinemia, and hypocalcemia. Diagnosis is largely based on a history of exposure and elimination of other causes of renal disease. Treatment is symptomatic, with diuresis and maintenance of electrolyte and acid-base balances being indicated.

Nephrotoxicity can also be induced by consumption of other plants. Ingestion of rayless goldenrod (*Isocoma wrightii*) may produce renal tubular nephrosis and signs of renal failure, but nephrotoxicity associated with this plant is uncommon. Tremetol is the most significant toxin present in the plant, and signs of toxicity are usually related to central nervous system depression and muscular dysfunction [7,8]. *Cestrum diurnum* (day-blooming jessamine, day cestrum, and wild jasmine) leaves contain a glycoside with potent vitamin D–like activity. Ingestion of this plant can result in dystrophic calcification of various soft tissues, including the kidney [3]. Wilted or dried red maple (*Acer rubrum*) leaves [9], hoary alyssum (*Berteroa incana*) [10], and onions (*Allium* spp) [3] can all cause hemolysis and subsequent pigment nephropathy attributable to excess hemoglobin (see the article by Schumacher elsewhere in this issue).

Treatment of these other plant-associated nephropathies is largely symptomatic. If plant-associated renal disease is suspected, the horse should be removed from the source as quickly as possible and suspect plants should be submitted for identification. Various state veterinary diagnostic laboratories, such as the Texas Veterinary Medical Diagnostic Laboratory (College Station, Texas), can be helpful in plant identification.

Medications

Aminoglycosides

Aminoglycoside toxicity in horses is almost exclusively manifested as nephrotoxicity, but neuromuscular blockade, direct myocardial depression, and eighth cranial nerve dysfunction have been described in human beings and other animal species [11].

Toxicity of aminoglycosides depends on several variables. Streptomycin is least nephrotoxic of the group; neomycin is most nephrotoxic; and amikacin, gentamicin, and kanamycin are intermediate in their ability to cause renal damage. The aminoglycosides are eliminated primarily by the kidney, and any cause of reduced renal blood flow or renal function can result in increased serum concentration of the drugs and increased potential for nephrotoxicity. Toxic potential is also increased by other factors, such as concurrent dehydration, hypovolemia, acidosis, endotoxemia, prolonged use of the drug, and increased dose or frequency of administration of the drug [3]. The concurrent use of other potentially nephrotoxic drugs, such as nonsteroidal anti-inflammatory drugs (NSAIDs) or oxytetracycline, may also predispose to aminoglycoside nephrotoxicity [11–15].

Diet may also influence the nephrotoxic potential of gentamicin, because horses fed oats had a greater degree of gentamicin-induced nephrotoxicity than did horses fed only alfalfa [16]. Concurrent intravenous administration of calcium has also been shown to attenuate gentamicin-induced acute renal failure in pony mares [17]. Low dietary calcium, potassium, and sodium have been shown to potentiate gentamicin-induced nephrotoxicity in laboratory animals, and increased dietary calcium demonstrated a protective effect against gentamicin-induced nephrotoxicity in rats [18].

Aminoglycosides are highly water soluble but poorly lipid soluble. They are rapidly absorbed from intramuscular and subcutaneous sites of injection [19,20] but are minimally absorbed from the intestinal tract. They are distributed essentially to the extracellular fluid space, and high concentrations of drug occur in the renal cortex [20,21]. Binding of drug to plasma proteins is minimal, and excretion occurs almost entirely by glomerular filtration of unchanged drug.

A small portion of filtered aminoglycoside accumulates within proximal tubular cells. This net reabsorption eventually results in high concentrations of drug within these cells, and, eventually, proximal tubular cell damage and death occur. With aminoglycoside nephrotoxicity, acute severe tubular necrosis rarely occurs and impaired renal function is almost always reversible because of the capacity of the proximal tubular cells to regenerate [3,20].

Aminoglycoside nephrotoxicity is manifested initially by evidence of proteinuria, cylindruria, polyuria, enzymuria, and hematuria. An increase in urinary gamma-glutamyl transferase (GGT) activity and the urinary GGT/creatinine ratio may be the earliest detectable laboratory changes noted with gentamicin toxicity and may precede increases in urinary protein and fractional clearance of phosphate by 48 hours [22]. Proteinuria and cylindruria may precede elevations in serum urea nitrogen and creatinine concentrations by several days [11,13]. From a practical standpoint, evaluating urine for the presence of increasing protein concentration seems to be a sensitive means of identifying early drug toxicosis.

Therapeutic drug monitoring can also be effective in decreasing the incidence of aminoglycoside nephrotoxicity, particularly in high-risk patients.

Measuring serum peak and trough concentrations of drug allows for individual dosage regimens suitable for each patient. Elevated trough values have been associated with increased incidence of nephrotoxicity and are more predictable indicators of toxicity than are serum peak concentrations. Optimal trough concentrations for aminoglycosides in horses have not been established; however, based on human guidelines, trough concentrations of less than 1 μg/mL for gentamicin and tobramycin and less than 2.5 μg/mL for amikacin are reasonably desired values [3].

Treatment of aminoglycoside nephrotoxicity usually involves adjustment of drug dosage (using therapeutic drug monitoring) or drug withdrawal, fluid diuresis, and urine alkalinization. In patients that require aminoglycoside therapy, reduced dosage or increased dosage interval may be required to minimize nephrotoxicity. Horses receiving moderate to large volumes of fluid usually have less than expected serum concentration of aminoglycoside when given at recommended dosages, and therefore rarely develop nephrotoxicity [3]. Additional treatments that can be used for aminoglycoside-induced nephrotoxicosis include peritoneal dialysis, plasmapheresis, and hemodialysis to reduce serum concentration of these drugs [23].

Sulfonamides

Historically, the sulfonamides have been incriminated as a cause of renal dysfunction but are now probably rarely involved in nephrotoxicity. Hematuria, crystalluria, and obstruction of renal tubules leading to anuria or tubular epithelial necrosis may occur after the administration of sulfonamides, especially when accompanied by low water intake and low urine pH [24]. The potentiated sulfonamides have much greater urine solubility and have not been incriminated as a cause of nephrotoxicosis in horses. Horses that are hypovolemic or have reduced renal function from other causes may be at greater risk for developing nephrotoxicosis than other horses.

Diagnosis is largely based on signs of acute renal failure accompanied by historical drug use and the presence of sulfonamide crystalluria. Treatment, if necessary, typically involves drug withdrawal, along with fluid diuresis and concurrent urine alkalinization.

Anecdotal reports of serious side effects after intravenous administration of potentiated sulfonamides may be associated with hypersensitivity, overdosage, or too rapid intravenous administration [24]. The combined use of intravenously administered trimethoprim-sulphadoxine with detomidine or halothane has also been associated with cardiac dysrhythmias, hypotension, and sudden death in several horses [24–26].

Oxytetracycline

A high dose (70 mg/kg of body weight administered intravenously) of oxytetracycline used to treat a neonatal foal with flexural limb deformity resulted in the foal developing acute renal failure [27]. Excessive doses of oxytetracycline have also been incriminated in producing nephrotoxicosis in calves [28] and dogs [29]. Other studies involving the intravenous administration of oxytetracycline to neonatal foals at doses ranging from 44 to 75 mg/kg of body weight given once or twice at a 24-hour interval did not result in signs or laboratory findings consistent with nephrotoxicity, however [30–32].

The high dose of oxytetracycline used to treat flexural limb deformity in neonatal foals may predispose some foals to tetracycline nephrotoxicosis. In calves and dogs, high doses of tetracyclines have been suggested to cause renal damage by inhibiting oxidative enzymes of tubular cells, with resultant hydropic degeneration and necrosis of the proximal tubular cells [28,29]. Also, propylene glycol, the vehicle for oxytetracycline, may decrease renal blood flow [27], and preexisting conditions, such as hypoxemia, hypovolemia, toxemia, septicemia, hemoglobinuria, myoglobinuria, and hyperbilirubinemia, and concurrent administration of nephrotoxic drugs may potentiate the toxicity of tetracyclines [27].

Diagnosis is suspected when clinical signs and laboratory findings consistent with acute renal failure are accompanied by historical use of large doses of oxytetracycline. Supportive and symptomatic care is required, because there is no specific treatment available.

Amphotericin B

Amphotericin B is a polyene antibiotic used to treat systemic fungal diseases in horses. It is a known nephrotoxin, and therapeutic and toxic levels of the drug overlap [3]. Amphotericin B causes direct injury to distal tubular epithelial cell membranes by combining with sterols on the lysosomal membranes of these cells. This allows for increased cell permeability, leakage of cytosol, and cell death [3]. Clinical signs of toxicity include anorexia, depression, weight loss, anemia (mild to severe), and fever. Extended use of the drug has also caused development of polyuria and polydipsia [3].

Diagnosis of toxicity is largely based on increasing blood urea nitrogen (BUN) concentration and urine findings of proteinuria, hematuria, and cylindruria [3]. An increase in BUN concentration greater than 40 to 50 mg/dL in human patients is cause for reduced dosage or temporary withdrawal of the drug [33]. Treatment involves fluid diuresis until the BUN concentration reaches a normal value. Nephrotoxicity caused by amphotericin B is reversible, and cessation of treatment usually results in return of renal function to almost normal levels. Additional therapies include the concomitant use of mannitol and oral sodium loading in an attempt to decrease the occurrence of azotemia [34].

Imidocarb dipropionate

Imidocarb dipropionate is an aromatic diamidine used as a chemotherapeutic agent for treatment of *Babesia equi* and *Babesia caballi* (piroplasmosis) in equids [35]. Current evidence suggests that four intramuscular

4-mg/kg doses of imidocarb dipropionate administered every 72 hours eliminate this red blood cell protozoan [35,36]. At this dosage, mild azotemia was reported in two of five horses, along with increases in urinary GGT activity and the urinary GGT/creatinine ratio [35]. Affected horses apparently returned to normal clinicopathologic indices after completion of the treatment regimen, and no other treatment was necessary.

Dose-dependent renal and liver toxicity have been attributed to this drug in various species, including dogs, goats, cattle, sheep, and horses [37]. In one study [37], increasing levels of imidocarb (16 or 32 mg/kg) were associated with increasing rates of morbidity and mortality attributed to acute renal cortical tubular necrosis and acute periportal hepatic necrosis. Other side effects noted with this drug relate to its anticholinesterase effects and include restlessness, salivation, hypermotility of the gastrointestinal tract, and colic. Local reactions varying from mild to severe at the injection site are common.

Vitamins D_2 and D_3

Most equine cases of vitamin D intoxication are iatrogenic, resulting from excessive use of vitamin supplements or from improperly formulated vitamin D–supplemented feeds. *C diurnum* (wild jasmine) contains a metabolically active glycoside of 1,25-dihydroxycholecalciferol, and ingestion of this plant can also result in vitamin D toxicosis.

Vitamin D_3 (cholecalciferol) is much more active and results in more severe lesions with wider tissue distribution than does an equivalent dose of vitamin D_2 (ergocalciferol) [3]. Duration of treatment and route of administration may also affect toxicosis, and increased concentrations of dietary calcium may enhance the effects of excessive amounts of vitamin D. The effect of vitamin D supplementation is cumulative, and signs of toxicity may not occur until weeks after supplementation has begun.

The toxicity of excessive amounts of vitamin D_3 results from extensive dystrophic mineralization rather than from any inherent toxicity of vitamin D itself. The most frequently affected soft tissue sites include the kidneys, tendons, and ligaments and the endocardium and walls of large blood vessels [3].

Clinical signs associated with vitamin D toxicosis are related to impairment of the renal, cardiovascular, or musculoskeletal system. Signs can include anorexia, depression, weakness, limb stiffness with impaired mobility, polyuria and polydipsia, cardiac murmurs and tachycardia, and recumbency. Calcification of tendons, ligaments, and other soft tissue structures may be palpable on physical examination [3].

Definitive diagnosis can be made by measuring serum concentrations of vitamins D_2 and D_3, and 1,25-dihydroxycholecalciferol. Other laboratory findings associated with toxicity can vary with the organ system affected but generally include pronounced and persistent hyperphosphatemia and hypercalcemia. The latter can vary daily, however, with serum calcium concentration remaining within a normal range in some horses. Other laboratory evidence of chronic renal failure may become evident with progression of toxicosis, and ultrasonographic evaluation of selected tissues may demonstrate abnormal mineralization within the tissues.

Treatment of vitamin D toxicosis should include removal of all exogenous sources of vitamin D. Recent evidence suggests that restricted feeding of calcium and phosphate should be initiated immediately once a diagnosis is made (or in the event of known administration of a toxic amount of vitamin D), because this may significantly reduce the amount of dystrophic calcification that may occur [38]. A cation chelator, such as sodium phytate, may be beneficial in reducing intestinal absorption of calcium, but the efficacy of this product has not been determined. Nonspecific treatment includes symptomatic therapy for renal insufficiency and failure, if necessary. Recovery may take months in less severely affected horses, but treatment is often unrewarding if excessive mineralization has occurred.

Menadione sodium bisulfite (vitamin K₃)

Vitamin K_3 causes acute renal failure in horses, but the product has been withdrawn from the US market [3]. When injected at the manufacturer's recommended dose of 2.2 to 11 mg/kg intravenously or intramuscularly, signs of toxicity became evident within 6 to 48 hours. Clinical signs of anorexia, depression, colic, hematuria, and stranguria were accompanied by laboratory findings of azotemia, electrolyte abnormalities, proteinuria, and isosthenuria. Pathologic lesions noted at necropsy were those of acute tubular necrosis, with one horse also showing renal interstitial fibrosis [3].

Treatment is symptomatic for acute or chronic renal failure.

Nonsteroidal anti-inflammatory drugs

NSAIDs are commonly used in equine veterinary practice. Although the gastrointestinal effects of NSAID toxicity are probably more common and more severe, renal damage attributable to these agents also occurs. Phenylbutazone seems to have the greatest toxic potential, followed by flunixin meglumine, with ketoprofen having the least toxic potential [39].

The real lesion typically associated with NSAID toxicity is medullary crest or papillary necrosis [3,40]. This lesion is associated with the inhibition of prostaglandin synthesis. Renal prostaglandins exert little control over basal renal blood flow in healthy animals, but in response to renal hypoperfusion, local production of the vasodilatory prostaglandins PGE_2 and PGI_2 is increased. The inhibition of prostaglandin synthesis by NSAIDs therefore results in decreased ability of the kidneys to autoregulate blood flow, leading to localized renal ischemia and necrosis [40,41]. Administration of NSAIDs to dehydrated or toxemic horses may further contribute to renal hypoperfusion by exacerbating a decrease in renal blood flow [3,40]. Additionally, foci of mineralization in the collecting tubules of the renal medullary region developed in 7- to 10-day-old foals that received phenylbutazone at a dosage of 5 mg/kg body weight orally twice daily for 7 days [42].

With chronic analgesic nephropathy, the area of papillary necrosis may serve as a nidus for nephrolith formation, and subsequent obstructive disease results in hydronephrosis [43].

NSAID toxicity should be suspected when compatible clinical signs are evident and the horse has a history of inappropriate drug administration. Hypoproteinemia and hypoalbuminemia are hallmarks of NSAID toxicity and are typically associated with gastrointestinal lesions. Indicators of renal dysfunction include increased concentrations of serum urea nitrogen, creatinine, and phosphorus, along with a mild decrease in total serum calcium concentration. Hematuria, macroscopic or microscopic, may be observed in the early stages of development of medullary crest necrosis. Transabdominal renal ultrasonography has revealed a hyperechoic outline of the corticomedullary junction, termed the *medullary rim sign* [44], in some horses (Fig. 1) and loss of normal renal pelvic architecture with medullary crest necrosis. Although the medullary rim sign is a remarkable ultrasonographic finding, it warrants emphasis that is it not specific for NSAID toxicity because it can also occasionally be found in horses with renal disease unassociated with NSAID use.

Treatment of analgesic nephropathy is largely symptomatic (see chapters 4 and 5 on acute renal failure and chronic renal failure, respectively). In affected horses, continued use of NSAIDs should be critically evaluated, and the drug(s) should be withdrawn if possible.

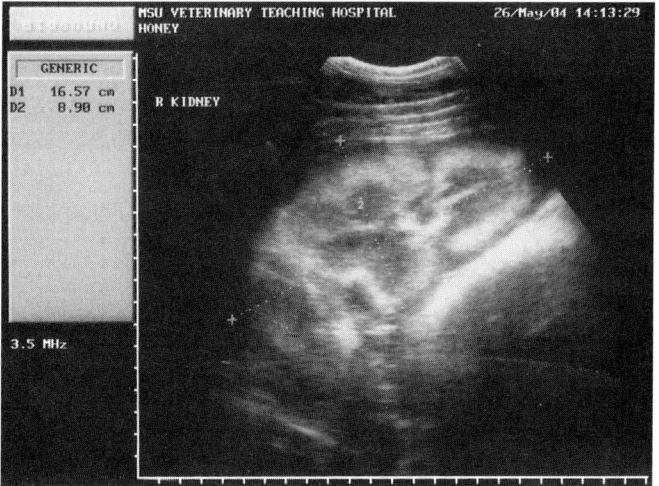

Fig. 1. Medullary rim sign in a 2-year-old quarter horse with acute laminitis and NSAID nephropathy. Note the increased echogenicity in the inner cortical region of the kidney surrounding the renal medulla. (*Courtesy of* H. Schott II, DVM, PhD, East Lansing, MI).

Miscellaneous agents

Mercury

Mercury exists in a variety of organic and inorganic forms, both of which can be toxic to horses [3,45]. The organic mercurial compounds are neurotoxic to central and peripheral nerves, with inorganic mercury salts being corrosive to the gastrointestinal tract. The absorbed fraction of inorganic mercurial salts is toxic to the kidneys [45].

Acute and chronic forms of toxicosis can occur in horses. The acute toxic dose of inorganic mercury in adult horses is 5 to 10 g [46]. Chronic inorganic mercury toxicity has been produced by ingestion of mercuric chloride at a dosage of 0.8 mg/kg/d over 14 weeks [47]. More recently reported cases of mercury toxicosis in horses have involved acute toxicity resulting from inorganic mercury-containing blistering agents applied topically to the skin [3,45,48].

Acute toxicity resulting from inorganic mercury can cause signs of acute renal failure, including oliguria and depression, and signs of gastrointestinal irritation. Excessive salivation, ulcerative stomatitis, abdominal pain, and diarrhea are common findings associated with gastrointestinal tract disturbances. Death can occur within hours to days after ingestion. Clinical signs of chronic intoxication with inorganic mercury include oral ulceration, anorexia, weight loss, alopecia, progressive respiratory difficulty, and terminal azotemia [3].

Inorganic mercury compounds are absorbed from the lungs and gastrointestinal tract and are poorly absorbed through the skin. After ingestion and absorption, mercury accumulates in the liver and kidneys, wherein it is concentrated to high levels within proximal renal tubular cells. Metallothionein binds mercuric ions within the endoplasmic reticulum of the tubular epithelial cells and then slowly releases mercury. The slow release of sequestered mercury can cause continued damage to tubular cells after the mercury source is removed. The development of mercury nephropathy is related to the amount of protein-bound mercury concentrated in the renal tubules. Bound mercury can remain in the kidneys for weeks after exposure. Acute toxicity results in massive tubular necrosis and acute renal failure, and chronic exposure may cause renal interstitial fibrosis leading to chronic renal failure [3].

Mercury intoxication should be suspected when horses show compatible clinical signs and lesions and have a history of exposure. Definitive diagnosis is usually based on measurement of mercury concentrations in blood, urine, and kidney and liver tissue. In renal tissue, more than 10 μg/g of mercury is considered diagnostic for acute mercury toxicity [46].

Treatment of mercury toxicosis must initially include removal of the source. In acute cases, evacuation of the bowel with mild laxatives and oral administration of activated charcoal (500 g) may be helpful. Further supportive care includes aggressive fluid therapy with correction of acid-base and electrolyte abnormalities, and chelation therapy may be attempted. No established regimen of chelation therapy for mercury exists in horses, but dimercaprol and N-acetyl-DL-penicillamine have been used. Dimercaprol can be given intramuscularly at a dosage of 3 mg/kg every 4 hours for the first 2 days, four times on the third day, and twice daily for the next 10 days until recovery is complete [49]. Penicillamine at a dose of 3 mg/kg administered orally every 6 hours was effective in increasing urinary excretion of mercury in one horse [48]. Treatment of chronic mercury intoxication is usually unrewarding.

Arsenic

Arsenic toxicosis in horses typically manifests as an acute syndrome. Because arsenic is efficiently excreted, chronic arsenic toxicity is rarely encountered. Sources of arsenic include certain herbicides and desiccants, wood preservative, and discontinued insecticides and rodenticides. Arsenic damages the gastrointestinal mucosa, resulting in necrotizing hemorrhagic typhlocolitis with necrotizing vasculitis. Arsenic also causes acute tubular nephrosis, but its effects on the gastrointestinal tract are of primary concern [45].

Clinical signs associated with acute inorganic arsenic toxicity in horses include salivation, trembling, ataxia, depression, abdominal pain, colic, diarrhea, and signs associated with severe shock. Death usually occurs within 12 to 24 hours of ingestion of a lethal dose. For horses, the average total oral lethal dose of arsenic trioxide is 10 to 45 g and that of sodium arsenite is 1 to 3 g [3]. Horses that survive may become azotemic and have laboratory findings compatible with renal dysfunction [45].

Definitive diagnosis of arsenic toxicosis is made by demonstrating more than 10 parts per million (ppm) arsenic in liver and kidney tissues. Horses surviving longer than 48 hours may have tissue concentrations in the 5- to 10-ppm range. Concentration of arsenic in urine can be determined antemortem to verify excessive exposure. Concentrations greater than 10 mg/L are indicative of excessive exposure [45].

Treatment of arsenic toxicosis is largely supportive. Additionally, sodium thiosulfate may be used to bind unabsorbed arsenic, and arsenic chelators, such as dimercaprol or D-penicillamine, may have beneficial therapeutic value [45].

Cadmium

Cadmium intoxication is rarely reported in horses but has been observed in animals living near smelting operations. Exposure usually results from grazing contaminated forage. Some urban sludges used as fertilizer may contain cadmium at a rate of 1500 ppm, and phosphate fertilizers may contain cadmium at a rate of 20 ppm. Both of these products are also potential sources of exposure to this metal. Acute toxicity attributable to cadmium is unlikely but can cause gastrointestinal signs of colic, anorexia, and diarrhea [3,45].

Usual clinical signs are those of unthriftiness, lameness, and swollen joints attributed to generalized osteochondrosis, osteoporosis, and nephrocalcinosis. Proteinuria is also reported in affected horses. With continued chronic exposure, renal fibrosis and atrophy may lead to chronic renal failure [3,45].

Diagnosis of chronic cadmium toxicosis is based on clinical signs of musculoskeletal dysfunction and nephrosis. Concentration of cadmium exceeding 100 ppm in liver and renal tissue is consistent with poisoning [45].

No specific treatment is established for chronic cadmium toxicity, and supportive care may be successful in rare cases of acute toxicosis [45].

Fumonisin

Fumonisins are mycotoxins produced by *Fusarium* fungi, primarily *Fusarium moniliforme*. This fungus is present in most all harvested corn, but toxin production is variable. Fumonisin B_1 is the principal toxin that causes mild to fatal disease in animals [50].

In horses, the most susceptible organ seems to be a function of dose. Higher doses are associated with brain lesions (leukoencephalomalacia), and lower doses more typically result in hepatotoxicity. Renal lesions caused by fumonisins are usually reported as incidental and have included hydropic degeneration, individual cell necrosis, and nephrosis [50]. Renal disease or dysfunction does not seem to be a significant aspect of fumonisin toxicosis in horses.

Summary

Many different substances can induce toxic damage to various structural components of the equine kidney, and most lack pathognomonic signs. Some of these agents have specific treatments, although many do not. Therefore, supportive and symptomatic therapy is an important aspect of treatment of most cases of equine nephrotoxicosis. Regardless of cause, if the toxic substance is removed or neutralized before significant renal damage, full recovery of renal function may occur. Many horses already have significant renal damage before a definitive diagnosis is made, however, and the prognosis for full recovery thus remains guarded.

References

[1] Adams LG, Dollahite JW, Romane WM, et al. Cystitis and ataxia associated with sorghum ingestion by horses. J Am Vet Med Assoc 1969;155(3):518–24.
[2] Van Kampen KR. Sudan grass and sorghum poisoning of horses: a possible lathyrogenic disease. J Am Vet Med Assoc 1970;156(5):629–30.
[3] Schmitz DG. Toxicologic problems. In: Reed SM, Bayly WM, Sellon DC, editors. Equine internal medicine. 2nd edition. St. Louis (MO): Saunders; 2004. p. 1441–512.

[4] Osweiler GD, Carson TL, Buck WB, et al. Oxalate. In: Clinical and diagnostic veterinary toxicology. 3rd edition. Dubuque (IA): Kendall/Hunt Publishing Company; 1985. p. 471–5.

[5] Hulbert LC, Oehme FW. Plants poisonous to livestock. 3rd edition. Manhattan (NY): Kansas State University; 1968. p. 35–8.

[6] Barr AC, Reagor JC. Toxic plants: what the horse practitioner needs to know. Vet Clin North Am Equine Pract 2001;17(3):529–46.

[7] Sperry OE, Dollahite JW, Hoffman GO, et al. Texas plants poisonous to livestock. Texas Agricultural Experiment Station Publication No. B-1028, College Station, Texas Agricultural Extension Service.

[8] Marsh CD, Roe GC, Clawson AB. Rayless goldenrod (*Aplopappus heterophyllus*) as a poisonous plant. Bulletin 1391. Washington, DC: US Department of Agriculture; 1926.

[9] Corriher CA, Parviainen AK, Gibbons DS, et al. Equine red maple leaf toxicosis. Compendium on Continuing Education for the Practicing Veterinarian 1999;21(1):74–80.

[10] Hovda LR, Rose ML. Hoary alyssum (*Berteroa incana*) toxicity in a herd of broodmare horses. Vet Hum Toxicol 1993;35(1):39–40.

[11] Riviere JE, Coppoc GL. Selected aspects of aminoglycoside antibiotic nephrotoxicosis. J Am Vet Med Assoc 1981;178(5):508–9.

[12] Schmitz DG. Toxic nephropathy in horses. Compendium on Continuing Education for the Practicing Veterinarian 1988;10(1):104–11.

[13] Riviere JE, Traver DS, Coppoc GLL. Gentamicin toxic nephropathy in horses with disseminated bacterial infection. J Am Vet Med Assoc 1982;180(6):648–51.

[14] Bartol JM, Divers TJ, Perkins GA. Case presentation: nephrotoxicant-induced acute renal failure in five horses. Compendium on Continuing Education for the Practicing Veterinarian 2000;22(9):870–6.

[15] Geor RJ. Case notes and commentary: drug-induced nephrotoxicity: recognition and prevention. Compendium on Continuing Education for the Practicing Veterinarian 2000; 22(9):876–8.

[16] Schumacher J, Wilson RC, Spano JS, et al. Effect of diet on gentamicin-induced nephrotoxicosis in horses. Am J Vet Res 1991;52(8):1274–8.

[17] Brashier MK, Geor RJ, Ames TR, et al. Effect of intravenous calcium administration on gentamicin-induced nephrotoxicosis in ponies. Am J Vet Res 1998;59(8):1055–62.

[18] Quarum ML, Houghton DC, Gilbert DN, et al. Increasing dietary calcium moderates experimental gentamicin nephrotoxicity. J Lab Clin Med 1984;103:104–14.

[19] Burrows GE. Aminocyclitol antibiotics. J Am Vet Med Assoc 1980;176(11):1280–1.

[20] Sande MA, Mandell GL, et al. Antimicrobial agents [continued]: aminoglycosides. In: Gilman AG, Goodman LS, Rall TW, editors. Goodman and Gilman's the pharmacological basis of therapeutics. 7th edition. New York: Macmillan; 1985. p. 1154–60.

[21] van der Harst MR, Bull S, Laffont CM, et al. Gentamicin nephrotoxicity—a comparison of *in vitro* findings with *in vivo* experiments in equines. Vet Res Commun 2005;29:247–61.

[22] Hinchcliff KW, McGuirk SM, MacWilliams PS. Gentamicin toxicity in pony mares. In: Proceedings of the Fifth Annual Veterinary Medical Forum (ACVIM). Madison (WI): Omnipress; 1987. p. 896.

[23] Divers TJ. Diseases of the renal system. In: Smith BP, editor. Large animal internal medicine. St. Louis (MO): Mosby-Year Book; 1990. p. 872–900.

[24] Van Duijkeren E, Vulto AG, Van Miert ASJPAM. Trimethoprim/sulfonamide combinations in the horse: a review. J Vet Pharmacol Ther 1994;17:64–73.

[25] Dick IGC, White SK. Possible potentiated sulphonamide-associated fatality in an anesthetized horse. Vet Rec 1987;121(12):288.

[26] Taylor PM, Rest RJ, Duckham TN, et al. Possible potentiated sulphonamide and detomidine interactions. Vet Rec 1988;122(6):143.

[27] Vivrette S, Cowgill LD, Pascoe J, et al. Hemodialysis for treatment of oxytetracycline-induced acute renal failure in a neonatal foal. J Am Vet Med Assoc 1993;203(1):105–7.

[28] Lairmore MD, Alexander AF, Powers BE, et al. Oxytetracycline-associated nephrotoxicosis in feedlot calves. J Am Vet Med Assoc 1984;185(7):793–5.

[29] Moalli MR, Dysko RC, Rush HG, et al. Oxytetracycline-induced nephrotoxicosis in dogs after intravenous administration for experimental bone labeling. Lab Anim Sci 1996; 46(5):497–502.

[30] Wright AK, Petrie L, Papich MG, et al. Effect of high-dose oxytetracycline on renal parameters in neonatal foals. In: Proceedings of the 38th Annual Convention of the American Association of Equine Practitioners. Lexington (KY): American Association of Equine Practitioners; 1992. p. 297–8

[31] Madson JB, Garber JL, Rice B, et al. Oxytetracycline decreases fetlock joint angle in newborn foals. In: Proceedings of the 38th Annual Convention of the American Association of Equine Practitioners. Lexington (KY): American Association of Equine Practitioners; 1992. p. 745–6.

[32] Madison JB, Garber JL, Rice B, et al. Effect of oxytetracycline on metacarpophalangeal and distal interphalangeal joint angles in newborn foals. J Am Vet Med Assoc 1994;204(2):246–9.

[33] Pyle RL. Clinical pharmacology of amphotericin B. J Am Vet Med Assoc 1981;179(1):83–4.

[34] Engelhardt JA, Brown SA. Drug-related nephropathies. II. Commonly used drugs. Compendium on Continuing Education for the Practicing Veterinarian 1987;9(3):281–8, 290.

[35] Meyer C, Guthrie AJ, Stevens KB. Clinical and clinicopathological changes in 6 healthy ponies following intramuscular administration of multiple doses of imidocarb dipropionate. J S Afr Vet Assoc 2005;76(1):26–32.

[36] Frerichs WM, Allen PC, Holbrook AA. Equine piroplasmosis (Babesia equi): therapeutic trials of imidocarb dihydrochloride in horses and donkeys. Vet Rec 1973;93:73–5.

[37] Adams LG. Clinicopathological aspects of imidocarb dipropionate toxicity in horses. Res Vet Sci 1981;31:54–61.

[38] Harmeyer J, Schlumbohm C. Effects of pharmacological doses of vitamin D_3 on mineral balance and profiles of plasma vitamin D_3 metabolites in horses. J Steroid Biochem Mol Biol 2004;89–90:595–600.

[39] MacAllister CG, Morgan SJ, Borne AT, et al. Comparison of adverse effects of phenylbutazone, flunixin meglumine, and ketoprofen in horses. J Am Vet Med Assoc 1993;202(1):71–7.

[40] Bayly WM. Acute renal failure. In: Reed SM, Bayly WM, Sellon DC, editors. Equine internal medicine. 2nd edition. St. Louis (MO): Saunders; 2004. p. 1221–30.

[41] MacAllister CG, Taylor-MacAllister C. Treating and preventing the adverse effects of nonsteroidal anti-inflammatory drugs in horses. Vet Med 1994;89(3):241–6.

[42] Leveille R, Miyabayashi T, Weisbrode SE, et al. Ultrasonographic renal changes associated with phenylbutazone administration in three foals. Can Vet J 1996;37:235–6.

[43] Schott HC II. Chronic renal failure. In: Reed SM, Bayly WM, Sellon DC, editors. Equine internal medicine. 2nd edition. St. Louis (MO): Saunders; 2004. p. 1231–53.

[44] Ramirez S, Seahorn TL, Williams J. Renal medullary rim sign in 2 adult quarter horses. Can Vet J 1998;39:647–9.

[45] Casteel SW. Metal toxicosis in horses. Vet Clin North Am Equine Pract 2001;17(3):529–46.

[46] Osweiler GD, Carson TL, Buck WB, et al. Organic and inorganic mercury. In: Clinical and diagnostic veterinary toxicology. 3rd edition. Dubuque (IA): Kendall/Hunt Publishing Company; 1985. p. 121–31.

[47] Roberts MC, Seawright AA, Ng JC, et al. Some effects of chronic mercuric chloride intoxication on renal function in a horse. Vet Hum Toxicol 1982;24(6):415–20.

[48] Guglick MA, MacAllister CG, Sundeep Chandra AM, et al. Mercury toxicosis caused by ingestion of a blistering compound in a horse. J Am Vet Med Assoc 1995;206(2):210–4.

[49] Schuh JCL, Ross C, Meschter C. Concurrent mercuric blister and dimethyl sulfoxide (DMSO) application as a cause of mercury toxicity in two horses. Equine Vet J 1988; 20(1):68–71.

[50] Bucci TJ, Howard PC, Tolleson WH, et al. Renal effects of fumonisin mycotoxins in animals. Toxicol Pathol 1998;26(1):160–4.

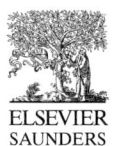

VETERINARY
CLINICS
Equine Practice

Vet Clin Equine 23 (2007) 691–696

ELSEVIER
SAUNDERS

Congenital Anomalies of the Equine Urinary Tract

Kristin P. Chaney, DVM

*Department of Large Animal Clinical Sciences, College of Veterinary Medicine,
Michigan State University, East Lansing, MI 48824–1314, USA*

Congenital anomalies of the urinary tract are rare in the horse but, when present, may be difficult to diagnose and treat. Presenting complaints are variable and include weight loss, depression, dysuria, hematuria, and mild colic, with the most severe anomalies presenting at earlier ages. Although most anomalies are diagnosed in the neonate, there are some diseases that are diagnosed in horses several months to years old. In human medicine, the fetus is examined before birth for evidence of urinary tract anomalies, but this is not yet common practice in equine medicine. As a result, urinary tract dysfunction is diagnosed after birth using a wide variety of diagnostic modalities.

The most common congenital anomaly of the equine urinary tract is ureteral ectopia. Ectopic ureter is diagnosed with greater frequency in fillies than in colts; in dogs, female animals are affected at a ratio of 8:1 with certain breed predispositions [1,2]. Ureteral ectopia occurs as a result of abnormal embryologic development of the metanephric bud. During organogenesis, the mesonephric duct develops a caudal outpouching, known as the metanephric bud, which advances in a cranial direction to interact with the metanephric blastema. It is the failure of the ureteric bud, or metanephric duct, to interact with the metanephric blastema that causes dysgenesis of the ureters, because the metanephric ducts develop into ureters bilaterally [3]. Failure of the metanephric bud to arise from its normal position on the mesonephric duct prevents the ureter from coursing normally into the dorsal bladder wall. Whether the metanephric bud arises medial or lateral from its normal position on the mesonephric duct, the ureter may empty into the uterus, vagina, or urethra [4]. Ureteral ectopia may be unilateral or bilateral; in dogs, approximately 25% are bilateral. Unilateral disease is most easily treated but may be more difficult to diagnose, because

---

E-mail address: chaneyk@cvm.msu.edu

doi:10.1016/j.cveq.2007.09.004   *vetequine.theclinics.com* these foals may be able to urinate a normal stream of urine. Depending on the location of the ectopia, urinary incontinence may or may not be observed with the classic sign of urine scalding of the perineum and hind limbs. Foals with an ectopic ureter have varying presenting complaints, because not all horses exhibit urinary incontinence. In fact, colts may be underdiagnosed with ectopic ureter because they are less likely to have evidence of urine scalding. Most often, renal function is normal in horses with ectopic ureter, without evidence of azotemia or systemic illness. In certain instances of bilateral disease, abnormalities of renal function may be observed, however, and in other cases of ureteral ectopia, additional congenital anomalies of the urinary tract may be present [5]. Whether or not urine scalding is observed, most foals, mainly fillies, exhibit some degree of urinary incontinence from birth but remain overtly healthy and capable of performing even the most intense athletic activity, such as race training [6]. Diagnosis is achieved using endoscopy, which allows direct visualization of the ectopic ureteral opening, with or without general anesthesia, depending on the size of the patient [6,7]. Endoscopy is facilitated with agents that discolor urine, such as azosulfamide or sodium fluorescein, to help define the location of ectopia [6]. Other diagnostic modalities that may facilitate diagnosis include ultrasonography and excretory pyelography [7]. More recently, the use of nuclear scintigraphy has been used to help define renal function in these horses before correction of the ectopia [8]. Before attempting correction, it is critical to determine whether disease is unilateral or bilateral, whether urinary tract infection (UTI) is present, whether the detrusor muscle has normal function, and whether the function of the renal system is intact. Once the location of the ectopia has been defined and the health of the contralateral kidney has been confirmed, several procedures exist for correction of the ectopic ureter. Ureteronephrectomy is an option but is contraindicated for bilateral disease. Ureteroneocystostomy is used for relocation of the ectopic ureter into its normal position within the dorsal bladder wall. Ectopic ureters may be dilated, however, making surgical manipulation difficult. In the past, there were reports of postoperative complications after surgical correction of ectopic ureters, including acute peritonitis and adhesion formation, which required the euthanasia of these surgical patients [9]. With the recent advancements in surgical techniques and development of equipment, such as the GIA50, however, greater success has been achieved with correction of ectopic ureters [8].

Failure of normal organogenesis of the ureters can lead to ureteral defects in addition to that of ureteral ectopia. Congenial ureteral defects consist of ureteral tears or rupture, ureteral atresia, and ureteropelvic junctional injuries (UPJs). Although foals with ectopic ureters seem otherwise healthy, foals with ureteral defects most commonly are presented with electrolyte abnormalities and azotemia, typical of a foal with a ruptured bladder or urachus [10]. These foals may also be presented at relatively younger ages (hours to days old) than are foals with ectopic ureters. Ureteral defects can cause urine leakage into the abdomen, leading to gross abdominal distention, or urine leakage into the retroperitoneal space, without evidence of uroperitoneum [11]. Diagnosis of uroperitoneum may be made by means of ultrasonography as black/anechoic fluid, combined with peritoneal paracentesis and a serum/peritoneal creatinine ratio of greater than 2:1 [12]. Failure to observe peritoneal fluid in a foal with hypochloremia, hyponatremia, hyperkalemia, and azotemia should prompt ultrasound examination of the retroperitoneal space, however. Additional tools useful to aid diagnosis include positive-contrast cystography, excretory urography, retrograde pyelography, and nuclear scintigraphy. Catheterization of the ureters retrograde from the bladder toward the renal pelvis using contrast material may be necessary to define the exact location of the ureteral defect(s) [13]. Although most ureteral defects are congenital, ureteropelvic junctional avulsion injury typically occurs after blunt trauma or accidental injury, as in human patients [14,15]. There is evidence to support underlying histopathologic findings of ureteral tissue, which allows the UPJ injury to occur, as in the case of a foal with UPJ after trauma from a dog attack [14,15]. After correction of the underlying systemic electrolyte imbalance that typically accompanies these foals, surgical intervention is required to correct the congenital defects. The use of ureteral stenting has been successful, with or without primary ureterorrhaphy. Other surgical procedures, such as ureteroneocystostomy, may be required depending on the degree of ureteral atresia [13]. Postoperative complications, including ureteral or urinary bladder catheter occlusion or complete failure of these catheters, rupture of the urinary bladder, ureteritis, leakage of urine around the suture material or stent, persistent anemia, and rerupture of the ureter(s), have all been reported [10–15]. These foals have a guarded prognosis, but if the repair is successful and the foal is discharged from the hospital, there are reports of long-term health of these individuals [12].

Other congenital anomalies of the urinary tract include renal hypoplasia and renal dysplasia. Renal dysplasia occurs because of abnormal nephrogenesis: the ureteric bud and the metanephric duct fail to interact normally [16]. When the ureteric bud arises from an abnormal position on the mesonephric duct, it is prevented from entering the center of the metanephrogenic blastema (embryonic renal parenchyma). Although contact with the periphery of the blastema may still result in the induction of a kidney, the induced renal tissue may be dysplastic. Although such a kidney may produce urine, it does not function normally [17]. The term *renal hypoplasia* results from dysplastic tissue; in human medicine, it is used to define greater than one third loss of total renal parenchyma and an overall lack of medullary tissue or in the case in which one kidney is less than 50% the size of the other [18,19]. The cause of parenchymal dysorganogenesis is unknown, even in people [19]. Although unilateral disease is most often reported, it may be because bilateral disease is incompatible with postnatal life. Unilateral hypoplasia typically leads to hypertrophy of the contralateral kidney with normal function, whereas bilateral renal hypoplasia results in chronic renal failure (CRF) [19]. Depending on the degree and severity of renal dysplasia, these foals may be presented from days to months old [20]. There are also reports of CRF related to renal hypoplasia found on routine blood work for elective procedures [21]. In patients that have renal hypoplasia or dysplasia, the clinical signs vary from weight loss and ill-thrift to diarrhea and depression [22]. Initial diagnosis of dysplastic kidneys includes blood work and evaluation of the urine. Azotemia and abnormal urinary fractional excretions of electrolytes (sodium, potassium, and chloride) and elevated gamma-glutamyltransferase (GGT)/creatinine ratios are typically observed [18]. Evaluation of the renal parenchyma may include ultrasonography, intravenous pyelography, CT, and ultrasound-guided renal biopsy. Dysplastic kidneys are typically small and misshapen, with poor corticomedullary distinction. Biopsy results may reveal immaturity of the glomeruli or tubules, with persistent mesenchyme and abnormal tubular epithelium, known as adenomatoid [20]. These histopathologic results are typical of renal biopsies from human dysplastic renal tissue. Although the kidneys are usually misshapen or difficult to identify, there is a report of a 2-day-old foal, presented with depression and diarrhea, with normal-sized kidneys and nearly normal numbers of glomeruli but with severe renal tubular hypoplasia that caused renal insufficiency [16]. In human patients, concurrent distal urinary tract obstruction of the ureter or urethra is often present with renal dysplasia. There is one such report in a 4-month-old Trakehner foal with hematuria and distal urinary tract obstruction [23]. A foal with bilateral dysgenesis of the kidneys with variable cortical development was also found to have concurrent ureteral involvement (ureteral atresia) at postmortem examination [24]. Although there are no reports of familial association of renal dysplasia in equine medicine, a genetic predisposition among Japanese black cattle has recently been shown [25].

Polycystic kidney disease is the fourth most common cause of renal failure in human medicine. This is an inherited, autosomal dominant, or recessive trait, and because most people present with clinical disease later in life, the trait is easily passed to offspring [3]. In veterinary medicine, polycystic kidney disease is also an autosomal dominant inherited trait with familial predispositions in long-haired and flat-faced cats. There is no such relation reported among horses, however. The cystic lesions grow slowly and begin to compress the surrounding parenchyma over time, leading to renal failure. Clinical signs are consistent with those of CRF: weight loss, depression, anorexia, and lethargy [26]. Diagnostic tests include blood work and ultrasound examination; there are no specific blood tests for hereditary disease in horses. Unfortunately, treatment is palliative only.

Another congenital anomaly involving the urogenital tract of foals is rectovaginal or rectourethral fistula. Because of the inherently related embryologic development of the caudal urogenital and gastrointestinal tracts, these two systems are interlinked. In the fetus, the gastrointestinal tract and urinary bladder terminate together into primitive cloaca. The urorectal septum arises and grows caudally, dividing the cloaca into dorsal (rectal) and ventral (urogenital sinus) portions. In the human fetus, the division of urogenital and rectal tissue should be complete by 46 days of gestation. Failure of the urorectal septum to divide the dorsal and ventral sinuses results in a persistent cloaca. Extrapolation from human studies on embryologic timing of division by the urorectal septum indicates that failure of septal formation in the horse probably occurs in the first trimester [27]. Failure of the septum to divide the cloaca results in a fistula between the urogenital tract and rectum or in more severe developmental failure, an imperforate anus. In male horses, the fistulous communication is most commonly seen between the rectum and the urethra, allowing feces to exit the urethra during urination, whereas in female horses, the fistula connects the rectum and the vagina [28]. These patients may be presented as young foals (<24 hours of age) but may also be months to years old. People are most often diagnosed later in life. Although the most common presenting complaints in these foals are UTI, hematuria, dysuria, and passage of urine through the anus, any foal born with atresia ani should be examined for a concurrent rectovaginal or rectourethral fistula [29]. Diagnosis of urogenital/rectal fistula in foals should include positive-contrast retrograde urethrography and radiographic study of the colon. Blood work on these individuals is typically nonreflective of urinary tract dysfunction (no azotemia or electrolyte imbalances related to renal insufficiency). In older horses, the fistula may be palpable by means of rectal examination and visualized by means of urethroscopy [30]. Treatment involves fistulectomy and additional rectoanoplasty for foals with atresia ani [29–31]. A heritable predisposition has been suspected for foals with atresia ani, and breeding these animals is not recommended [31].

References

[1] Ureteral anomalies: ectopic ureter. In: Kahn CM, Line S, editors. Merck veterinary manual. 9th edition. Whitehouse Station: Merck & Co., Inc.; 2005. p. 1254.
[2] Holt PE, Thrusfield MV, Moore AH. Breed predisposition to ureteral ectopia in bitches in the UK. Vet Rec 2000;146:561.
[3] Welling LW, Grantham JT. Cystic and developmental diseases of the kidney. In: Brenner BR, Rector FC, editors. The kidney. 3rd edition. Philadelphia: WB Saunders Co; 1986. p. 1341–76.
[4] Schott HC II. Disorders of the urinary system. In: Reed SM, Bayly WM, Sellon DC, editors. Equine internal medicine. 2nd edition. St. Louis: Saunders; 2004. p. 1169–83.
[5] Houlton JEF, Wright IM, Matic S, et al. Urinary incontinence in a Shire foal due to ureteral ectopia. Equine Vet J 1987;19(3):244–7.
[6] MacAllister CG, Perdue BD. Endoscopic diagnosis of unilateral ectopic ureter in a yearling filly. J Am Vet Med Assoc 1990;197(5):617–8.
[7] Blikslager AT, Greene EM, MacFadden KE, et al. Excretory urography and ultrasonography in the diagnosis of bilateral ectopic ureters in a foal. Vet Radiol Ultrasound 1992;33(1): 41–7.
[8] Gettman LM, Ross MW, Elce YA. Bilateral ureterocystostomy to correct left ureteral atresia and right ureteral ectopia in an 8-month-old Standardbred filly. Vet Surg 2005;34:657–61.

 [9] Modransky PD, Wagner PC, Robinette JD, et al. Surgical correction of bilateral ectopic ureters in two foals. Vet Surg 1983;12(3):141–7.
[10] Divers TJ, Byars TD, Spirito M. Correction of bilateral ureteral defects in a foal. J Am Vet Med Assoc 1988;192(3):384–6.
[11] Robertson JT, Spurlock GH, Bramlage LL, et al. Repair of ureteral defect in a foal. J Am Vet Med Assoc 1983;183(7):799–800.
[12] Jean D, Marcoux M, Louf C-F. Case report: congenital bilateral distal defect of the ureters in a foal. Equine Vet Educ 1998;10(1):17–20.
[13] Morisset S, Hawkins JF, Frank N, et al. Surgical management of a ureteral defect with ureterorrhaphy and of ureteritis with ureteroneocystostomy in a foal. J Am Vet Med Assoc 2002;220(3):354–8.
[14] Cutler TJ, MacKay RJ, Johnson CM, et al. Bilateral ureteral tears in a foal. Aust Vet J 1997; 85(6):413–5.
[15] Kawashima A, Sandler CM, Corriere JN Jr, et al. Ureteropelvic junction injuries secondary to blunt abdominal trauma. Radiology 1997;205:487–92.
[16] Zicker SC, Marty GD, Carlson GP, et al. Bilateral renal dysplasia with nephron hypoplasia in a foal. J Am Vet Med Assoc 1990;196(12):2001–5.
[17] Hatch DA. Genitourinary development: a tutorial correlating embryology with congenital anomalies. David A. Hatch, M.D. Professor of Urology & Pediatrics, Loyola University Stritch School of Medicine. 1996 (Internet tutorial).
[18] Gull T, Schmitz DG, Bahr A, et al. Renal hypoplasia and dysplasia in an American miniature foal. Vet Rec 2001;149:199–203.
[19] Maxie MG. The urinary system. In: Jubb KVF, Kennedy PC, Palmer N, editors. Pathology of domestic animals, vol. 2. 3rd edition. San Diego (CA): Academic Press; 1985.
[20] Anderson WI, Picut CA, King JM, et al. Renal dysplasia in a standardbred colt. Vet Pathol 1988;25:179–80.
[21] Ramierez S, Williams J, Seahorn TL, et al. Ultrasound-assisted diagnosis of renal dysplasia in a 3-month old QH colt. Vet Radiol Ultrasound 1998;39(2):143–6.
[22] Andrews FM, Rosol TJ, Kohn CW, et al. Bilateral renal hypoplasia in four young horses. J Am Vet Med Assoc 1986;189(2):209–12.
[23] Jones SL, Langer DL, Sterner-Kock A, et al. Renal dysplasia and benign ureteropelvic polyps associated with hydronephrosis in a foal. J Am Vet Med Assoc 1994;204(8):1230–4.
[24] Brown CM. Bilateral renal dysplasia and hypoplasia in a foal with an imperforate anus. Vet Rec 1988;122:91–2.
[25] Ohba Y, Kitagawa H, Kitoh K, et al. Inheritance of renal tubular dysplasia in Japanese Black cattle. Vet Rec 2001;149:115–8.
[26] Aguilera-Terjero E, Estepa JC, Lopez I, et al. Polycystic kidneys as a cause of chronic renal failure and secondary hypoparathyroidism in a horse. Equine Vet J 2000;32(2):167–9.
[27] Furie WS. Persistent cloaca and atresia ani in a foal. Equine Practice—Medicine 1983;5(1): 30–3.
[28] Kingston RS, Park RD. Atresia ani with associated urogenital tract anomaly in foals. Equine Practice 1982;4(1):32–4.
[29] Chandler JC, MacPhail CM. Congenital urethrorectal fistulas. Compendium 2001;23(11).
[30] Cruz AM, Barber SM, Kaestner SB, et al. Urethrorectal fistula in a horse. Can Vet J 1999; 40(2):122–4.
[31] Jansson N. Anal atresia in a foal. Equine Rounds—Compendium November: 2002;888–90.

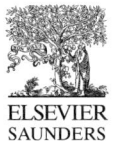

ELSEVIER
SAUNDERS

Vet Clin Equine 23 (2007) 697–701

VETERINARY
CLINICS
Equine Practice

Index

Note: Page numbers of article titles are in **boldface** type.

Moving?

Make sure your subscription moves with you!

To notify us of your new address, find your **Clinics Account Number** (located on your mailing label above your name), and contact customer service at:

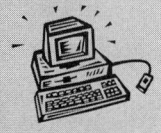

E-mail: elspcs@elsevier.com

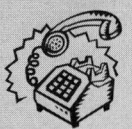

800-654-2452 (subscribers in the U.S. & Canada)
407-345-4000 (subscribers outside of the U.S. & Canada)

Fax number: 407-363-9661

Elsevier Periodicals Customer Service
6277 Sea Harbor Drive
Orlando, FL 32887-4800

*To ensure uninterrupted delivery of your subscription, please notify us at least 4 weeks in advance of move.

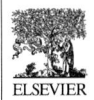